Understanding
Three-Dimensional Images
Recognition of Abdominal Anatomy from CAT Scans

Computer Science:
Artificial Intelligence, No. 13

Harold S. Stone, Series Editor

Professor of Electrical and Computer Engineering
University of Massachusetts, Amherst

Other Titles in This Series

Understanding Three-Dimensional Images

Recognition of Abdominal Anatomy from CAT Scans

by
Uri Shani

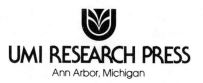

UMI RESEARCH PRESS
Ann Arbor, Michigan

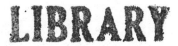

Produced and distributed by
UMI Research Press
an imprint of
University Microfilms International
Ann Arbor, Michigan 48106

Library of Congress Cataloging in Publication Data

Shani, Uri.
  Understanding three-dimensional images.

  (Computer science. Artificial intelligence ; no. 13)
  Revision of thesis (Ph.D.)–University of Rochester,
1981.
  Bibliography: p.
  Includes index.
  1. Abdomen–Anatomy. 2. Abdomen–Radiography.
3. Tomography. I. Title. II. Series.

QM543.S5 1983   611'.95   83-15818
ISBN 0-8357-1521-3

To Zipi, Guy, and Erez

Contents

List of Tables and Listings

List of Figures

Acknowledgments

I am grateful for the superb supervision and guidance of my advisor Dana Ballard: for the lengthy discussions, the useful suggestions, and, in particular, for the deep optimism and belief in the success of this work that he shared with me in a very friendly way. I am also thankful to those numerous people in the Computer Science Department of the University of Rochester who contributed software that was necessary to develop this study, and for their suggestions, criticism, and encouragement. The members of the Radiology Department in Strong Memorial Hospital aided me in selecting and acquiring data—in particular Derek Hamlin.

In preparing this text, special thanks to Peggy Meeker and Rose Peet for help in the initial stages. The Nondestructive Evaluation (NDE) Program at General Electric Corporate Research and Development has given me the means and time for the final editing of the manuscript, which was supervised by Catharine L. Fisher for whose dedicated and professional work I am very grateful.

Some of the mathematical contributions of this study were aided by the MACSIMA system at the Massachusetts Institute of Technology, Boston, to which I had access via the ARPANET. Also I thank Klaus Gradischnig for his help in translating an article written in German.

I am grateful to the members of my Ph.D. committee, who have read several versions of this study, and provided me with useful comments and guidance in the overall writeup, organization, and contents, each in his spcialized field: Gershon Kedem in mathematics, Chris Brown in geometric modeling and AI, and Don Plewes in radiology and medicine.

This work could not have been achieved if it had not been for the support and care of my beloved parents, who made available to me the necessary and appropriate background. Last and dearest, thanks to my loving and patient wife, Zipi, and my sons, Guy and Erez, who helped me come through, hoping (with me) for the good days lying ahead.

Thank you all.

This work was supported in part by National Institutes of Health grant R23-HL-21253.

Foreword

Machine analysis and understanding of three-dimensional (3-D) images is a relatively new field compared to the conventional image analysis of two dimensions (2-D) only. Surprising as it may seem, humans are not well equipped to visualize 3-D *images,* although in fact they do very well with 3-D *scenes,* of which a 2-D projection is analyzed and understood by the human intelligence. This fact is a major motivation for research in the area of 2-D machine vison, since if one understands well enough the human visual processes, one may design computerized systems with similar performance. In fact, some of the more successful image analysis techniques utilize human-based models. CAT scans provide an example of a 3-D image which is commonly viewed as a set of 2-D slices. Medical CAT scans exhibit many favorable attributes for a model-driven (knowledge-based) approach, besides being practical and nontrivial. A comparably favorable domain would have

This study presents the background, motivations, and details of a model-driven system for analyzing such 3-D images, examples of its behavior and results, and a comparison of this approach with other projects in this area and in closely related areas. The study is organized in two parts: the *main text* of six chapters and eight *appendices* of supplementary and complementary material. Of the main chapters, the first two are introductory and general discussions, the middle two are technical, and the last two are summaries. Of the appendices, Appendix A is a general background, Appendices B, D, F, G, and H are technical complements to the main text, and Appendices C and D are additional examples.

Chapter 1 describes the rationale for a model-driven approach by providing an appropriate perspective of 3-D CAT images and presenting the short- and long-range benefits of this approach. Appendix A relates to this chapter.

Chapter 2 surveys various modeling techniques and previous uses of the chosen tool, the Generalized-Cylinder. It also presents the definition of an extended Generalized-Cylinder using parametric uniform cubic B-splines. Both Appendices B and F relate to this chapter.

Chapter 3 presents a description of the strategy for fitting a model-instance to data in a hierarchical manner, via the hierarchical model structure, and explains the role of *experts*.

Chapter 4 portrays the details of implementing and applying the techniques presented in Chapter III, using the SAIL programming language. In this context, the experts used for recognizing the kidney in abdominal CAT images are discussed.

Chapter 5 depicts three levels of examples, in one, two, and three dimensions.

Chapter 6 summarizes and concludes the achievements, failures, and shortcomings of this work, and outlines prospects for future research. Other projects in 3-D image analysis are compared.

In the appendices:

Appendix A provides technical background for CAT scans.

Appendix B presents technical background for B-splines, and some new techniques for manipulating uniform cubic parametric B-spline curves.

Appendix C is a pretty-print of a portion of the internal model representation.

Appendix D describes the methods and procedures used to acquire CAT data, and the organization of multiresolution, 3-D images.

Appendix E is an addition to Chapter 5 (examples), in listing a detailed, step-by-step trace of the 3-D fitting process, including timing.

Appendix F is a technical addition to the mathematics involved in the definition of Generalized-Cylinders in Chapter 2.

Appendix G is a background introduction to SAIL and LEAP environments, and a discussion of the alternatives for knowledge representation as used in the model definition.

Appendix H is an overview of the implemented system with its components and organization.

1

Introduction

1.1 Two-Dimensional and 3-D Image Analysis

Research in machine understanding of 2-D images is rich in analogies from natural visual processes and systems. Most notable are algorithms for the detection of edges in images: the Hough transformation [Hough, 1962], Hueckel operator [Hueckel, 1969], or the simpler gradient operator [Duda & Hart, 1973]. These techniques were influenced by the discovery of the so-called "receptive fields" of neuron cells along the visual path [Hubel & Wiesel, 1962]. Neuron cells were found to be sensitive not only to edges in the retinal image but also to spatial frequencies in it. Such are the "complex" cells that were discovered in the cat cerebral cortex by Hubel and Wiesel. Fourier analysis of the spatial frequencies in images, though already well practiced at that time, has been even more encouraged by this discovery. Research in human color perception added another dimension to image analysis by introducing the "opponent color theory" [Hering, 1961]. This theory was used in analyzing pictures of outdoor scenes [Sloan; Sloan & Bajcsy, 1977]. Other experiments in explaining human recognition of images introduced the theory of "primal sketch" [Marr & Nishihara, 1977], and the use of "stick figures" to model animals in pictures and guide an automatic recognition system [Marr & Nishihara, 1976].

The analogy from natural vision to machine vision is quite intuitive; the computer is presented with an image that is a projection of a scene on a viewing-plane, which is then "sampled" to provide numerical representations of some attributes of "pixels," small rectangular pieces of the picture. This process is similar to what happens in the very first stage of natural vision: the excitation of receptor cells in the retina by the light intensity and spectral contents of small pieces of the retinal image which is the projection of a scene. This very close relation between a scene and its image in natural vision and images formed by machine representation (raster images) is depicted in Figure 1.1. If the image created on the retina is understood by humans, there is hope that similar performance is achievable from a computer.

Figure 1.1   There is a close relation between a retinal image and
an electronically digitized raster image.

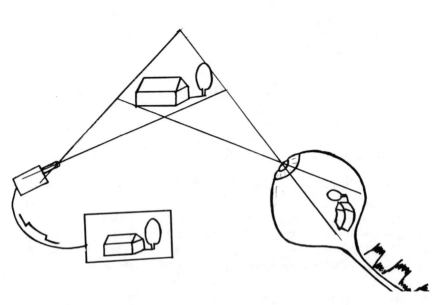

The relation between a scene and its image in the 3-D case is totally different from a 2-D case. Clearly, there is no similar phenomenon in nature. A 3-D image represents some attributes of the material in a *finite* volume that occupies the scene. More accurately, each element of the 3-D image samples a corresponding parallelepipe small volumetric piece (termed *voxel*) of the scene by representing, say, the material density there. When such an image is mathematically projected (i.e., by integration of all the values along projection lines) on a plane, the created 2-D image resembles a radiograph of the scene. Figure 1.2 pictures a comparison between the relations of a 3-D scene to its two- and three-dimensional images.

Three-dimensional images are created by various means: ultrasonic imagery [Greenleaf, 1979; Havlice, 1979] of either B-scans or ultrasonic CT scans [Mueller, 1979], electron microscopy [Gilbert, 1972], CAT scans [Hounsfield, 1972], Nuclear Magnetic Resonance (NMR) imaging [Hinshaw, 1983], radio astronomy [Bracewell, 1956] (though he was interested in 2-D reconstruction only), geology [Dines, 1979], and others.

The technique used in most of these cases is called "Reconstruction from Projections" [Herman, 1980] and is based on the, already classic, work of [Radon, 1917] that when infinitely many projections (integrations) are given along straight lines through a space (2 or 3 dimensions) in which a continuous function, F, is defined, that function may be reconstructed. When the number

Figure 1.2   The relationship between a radiograph and
computerized tomography. While the radiograph is a
projection of the image on a plane, the computerized
tomograph (only one slice shown) provides a
numerical value for each volumetric voxel in the
scene. (From "Image Reconstruction from
Projections" by Richard Gordon, Gabor T. Herman
and Steven A. Johnson,©1975 by *Scientific American,*
Inc., all rights reserved.)

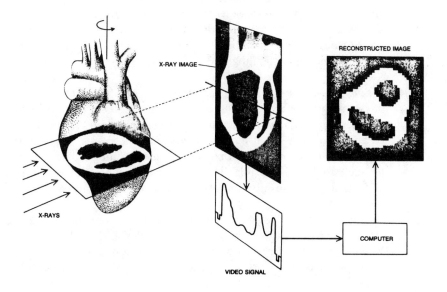

of such projections is only finite, then only a discrete approximation to the
function F is achieved [Gordon, 1974].

The differences between 2- and 3-dimensional images introduce new
problems while eliminating others. These differences in respect to 2-D image
analysis range from the relation between a scene and its image to the drastically
increased amount of data in 3-D images. Some of these differences are
described below.

1. *Scene-image relations:* As depicted in Figure 1.2, there is much more
    explicit information in 3-D images; thus some of the most difficult
    problems in 2-D image analysis, such as occlusion and the ambiguity
    of scene-image relations, are eliminated. The scene is of a finite size,
    and no projection distortion affects the image, which is a sample of the
    volume that occupies the scene; thus high spatial detail in 3-space is
    provided.

2. *Human visualization:* Two-dimensional images are easy to visualize, which is not true for 3-D images. In this case, one must distinguish between the 3-D image and its 3-D scene, since one has no problem understanding a 3-D scene (if one could only see what is inside).

3. *Human vision analogy:* Machine analysis of 2-D images has been greatly influenced by research in human vision, since there is a strong analogy between the human imagery process in the retina and the computer digitization of pictures (Figure 1.1). There is not, however, any process in nature parallel to 3-D imaging, for instance with a CAT-scanner. If the human retina were three-dimensional, perhaps some analogies could have been made between a human vision system and machine understanding of 3-D images.

4. *Model as a basis for understanding:* Any successful system for 2-D image analysis [Hanson, 1978] is based on some kind of a model to represent some knowledge about the scene. This model is frequently based on a theory about human visual mental processes, i.e., there is an effort to make analogies. In machine understanding of 3-D images, no such analogy is feasible. The geometry of scanned objects is an important source of information for modeling the scene.

5. *Amount of data:* Three-dimensional images have more data than 2-D images. The data will increase with more advanced CAT-scanners. When presented with such an increase in the amount of raw data, many methods that work well for 2-D will become computationally impractical.

1.2 Computed Axial Tomographs: Three-Dimensional Images

Computed Axial Tomography (CAT) for medical purposes is the area that makes the greatest use of the technique of reconstruction from projections. CAT scans are naturally associated with this application that came into being when the first CAT-scanner was built by the EMI Corporation [Hounsfield, 1972]. This invention is considered one of the most important discoveries in medicine since 1895, when Wilhelm Konard Roentgen discovered the X-ray. The principles and history of medical CAT scanning are presented in Appendix A. Today, the CAT-scanner is an essential piece of equipment in any modern hospital in the country. Although CAT scanning has been predominantly associated with medical applications, this is currently changing. Computer Axial Tomograms will play an important role in many other fields, such as non-destructive testing in manufactured parts inspection.

Figure 1.3   A CAT scan is a set of 2-D slides, which when
stacked , comprise a 3-D image. This photograph
(originally made on ordinary X-ray plates) consists of
18 CAT slices which "cover" a volume that contains
the two kidneys. This can serve as one of the data sets
on which this thesis was tested.

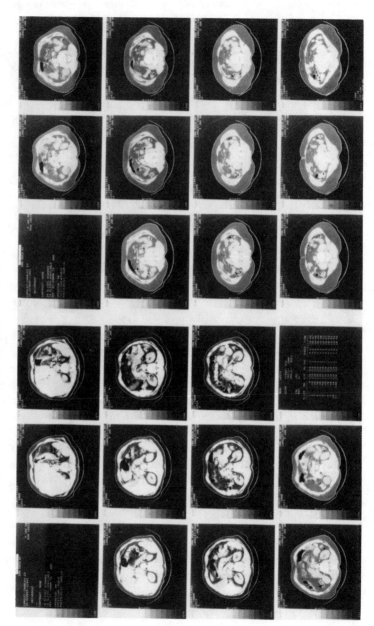

Figure 1.4   A 3-D shaded image of three organs: the two kidneys
and part of the spinal column. This kind of organ
display is an expected result of this thesis.

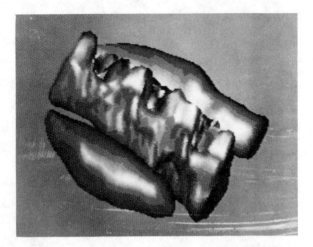

Despite the fact that most CAT-scanners work plane-wise [Brooks, 1975] and provide the image as a stack of cross sections (slices), each a 2-D image (see Figure 1.3), it is more appropriate to perceive the image as a three-dimensional array of which each element samples the linear attenuation coefficient for X-ray absorption of the material in a corresponding voxel in the scene. Current research in this area concentrates on the rapid reconstruction of 3-D images directly, without going through the 2-D intermediate stage. Mathematical background is given in [Altschuler, 1979], and a working prototype in the Mayo Clinic in Rochester, Minnesota, is designed to provide a direct 3-D image of high resolution and at a very high speed [Riteman, 1979].

To examine a CAT scan, a diagnostician can view the slices, and other arbitrary cross sections of the 3-D image, that may be mathematically interpolated [Klinger, 1979]. These views are limited to 2-D and do not reveal the full potential of the 3-D image. A 3-D representation of objects that are in the scene is preferred. Once the 3-D representation of objects is found, it can be displayed by computer-graphics techniques, thus revealing the information in the image to its fullest extent. Three-dimensional image analysis is regarded here as the generation of such a representation.

Besides improving the visual quality of 3-D images, the 3-D geometric representation of objects in the scene may serve a large range of quantitative applications:

1. Provide geometrical measurements such as volume, surface area, and mass;

2. Pinpoint defects in production of industrial parts by comparing the recovered 3-D geometry with the original design of scanned objects; and

3. Serve as a valuable source of statistical studies in medicine, of the anatomical geometry of humans and other species. It may automate the analysis of medical CAT scans, as well as some of their other applications.

As mentioned before, this study concentrates on the analysis of medical CAT images.

1.3 Approaches to 3-D Image Analysis

Of the large varieties of approaches to this problem, a very popular one is to outline (manually) the boundaries of an object as seen at each intersecting plane (slice). This outline is digitized as a set of contours to serve for 3-D computer-graphic display [Fuchs, 1977], or wire-frame graphic animation [Cohen, 1978]. In a different application, the volume, mass, and center of gravity of human organs were measured based on a manual contour-following technique for processing CAT images [Huang, 1980]. This tedious approach can be automated by applying 2-D image analysis techniques to each of the 2-D slices in the 3-D image. Rhodes utilized a "region growing" technique that worked slice-wise, but examined each slice several times to determine the object geometry in an attempt to minimize the number of slice-reentries [Rhodes, 1979]. Elsewhere, Selfridge tried to locate a cross section of the kidney in a planar CAT scan, as a problem in 2-D image analysis [Selfridge, 1979]. Also worth mentioning is the important work of Soroka, who viewed the problem as "understanding objects from slices" [Soroka, 1979; 1981]. Soroka tried to locate 3-D objects by fitting conics to image features of individual CAT slices, and to combine them to create "Generalized-Cones" (hereafter referred to as Generalized-Cylinders, or shortly, GC's [Agin, 1972]) for the representation of 3-D objects (see also discussion in Chapter 2).

A direct approach to analyzing the image as a 3-D structure, without any bias toward its slice-wise acquisition process, was first reported in [Liu, 1977]. Liu implemented a 3-D boundary-following algorithm to recover the boundary surface of objects. This approach is challenging, since it tries to use, in higher dimensions, methods which have only been well-practiced in 2-D image analysis (see also [Herman, 1978]). In this method, discovered objects are represented as the collection of all found voxels, on their boundaries, and are then displayed by means of pseudo 3-D graphics [Herman, 1979]. The extension of 2-D edge operators into the 3-D world has also been reported in [Zucker, 1979], where CAT images are searched as 3-D images *per se,* and tiny planar facets are detected at the center of voxels, by a 3-D analogy of the 2-D Hueckel operator [Hueckel, 1971].

1.4 Image and Scene Attributes in Medical CAT Scans

All the approaches mentioned above are general enough to operate on any kind of 3-D image. The fact is, however, that they have been mostly applied to CAT scans, and particularly for medical applications. Medical CAT scans display some important attributes for both the image and its scene that together serve as an important incentive to achieve a different, domain-specific approach.

1.4.1 Image Attributes

Image attributes are mainly the 3-D characteristics of the image, but they are also the quantitativeness of CAT numbers.

1. *Direct 3-D sample of the scene:* Every voxel in the scene is represented in the image by the average linear attenuation coefficient of X-ray absorption of the material in it, termed the *CAT number.* The correspondence between image elements and voxels in the scene provides an accurate representation of 3-D spatial information about the scene.

2. *Quality and quantitativeness:* CAT scanning is a well-controlled process taken under well-observed conditions. CAT image quality is high compared to other 3-D imaging techniques (e.g., ultrasonics), but CAT images suffer from artifacts and low resolution compared to regular X-ray (refer to Appendix A for technical details). However, CAT images are superior to any of the other techniques (2-or 3-D) in being highly quantitative, thus providing some means to correlate CAT numbers with material types in their corresponding voxels.

1.4.2 Anatomical Scene Attributes

These are the spatial relations, geometry, and tissues of the set of organs (objects) in the scene. The main three attributes are (cf. Figs. 2.1, 2.2 below):

1. Organs have typical shapes, on which most of us base our recognition of them: a longitudinal axis that is typical of the various organs and a smooth surface that they usually have;

2. Gross anatomy is well structured in that organs have typical locations, and relate spatially in a way that is common to all humans (e.g., all scenes); and

3. Classes of organs have their typical range of tissue types which correspond to quantitative CAT numbers.

The quantitative nature of CAT numbers is a controversial issue. Although calculated by means of a precise mathematical algorithm, CAT numbers are affected by many parameters which are patient- and scanning-dependent. The patient's parameters are his health, age, sex, size, and medical history. Scanning parameters are machine-dependent; they depend also on the type of contrast agent taken by the patient prior to the scan. The relationship between some of these factors and the correlation between CAT numbers and tissue types are reported in [Mategrano, 1977], while in [Plewes, 1980] we can find a survey of efforts to use contrast material uptake as an aid in tumor diagnosis. Although Mategrano concluded that there is no clear-cut correlation between CAT numbers and specific organ tissues, there is some correlation between *groups* of tissues (e.g., bones, fat, and muscles) and ranges of CAT numbers. Also, within the data for a single patient, there is an apparent change in CAT numbers for neighboring tissues (those that define boundaries in a CAT image) that is correlated to tissue types. In [Huang, 1980], the correlation between CAT numbers and tissues is used to compute organ mass, center of mass, and moments, following a manual outline of tissue boundaries in CAT slices. We feel that there has not been enough empirical study (probably due to its complexity) of how we can infer from a given set of external parameters the relationship between CAT numbers and tissue types. Obviously, for the purpose of image analysis, a successful prediction system to infer the relation of CAT numbers to neighboring organs is extremely useful. The difficulties of correlating specific organs to distinguished CAT numbers (as concluded by Mategrano) do not ban the usefulness of quantitative CAT numbers.

The intent of using quantitative CAT numbers is not to threshold an image, thus simplifying the "extraction" of objects' shapes,* but to distinguish the types of boundaries between an interesting organ and its surroundings. This study provides the tools for using such knowledge; it contends that the more precise and available the knowledge, the more successful will be a model-driven system in extracting organ shapes in CAT images, although the quantitativeness of CAT numbers is used only limitedly across organ boundaries.

Knowledge of typical shapes and sizes of organs is important mostly for an appropriate anatomy modeling, and is considered essential for numerous medical diagnosis purposes. CAT scans have been used extensively in medical research to support organ contour tracing, such as that done by Mategrano et al. (see also references for studies of organ shapes from CAT scans in [Kuo, 1979]). Kuo and his colleagues have tried to build a computerized data-base of organ sizes and shapes for comparative purposes, based on an initial collection of 60 cases. The existence of such data-bases and an automatic CAT analyzing system, such as described in this study, will have substantial mutual benefits. To make this relation more fruitful, the correspondence between organs' shape parameters and patient parameters should be studied (as suggested for the utilization of CAT numbers).

1.5 Approach and Technical Contributions

Most of the approaches to the problem until now were data-driven. That is, a local operator is applied to the data and, based on few adjacent voxels, it responds strongly if there is evidence of an object boundary. The results of the exhaustive application of the operator are then combined into notions of objects. These approaches are easily hindered by noisy data but work well where the effects of noise are negligible; this is true with the systems of Liu and of Rhodes, which perform splendidly for the detection of bone tissues and the lungs—cases where boundary detection is decisive. The difficulties of using a data-driven approach to evaluate noisy data are discussed by Selfridge [1979], who attempts to tackle the problem of automatically outlining the kidney, a soft organ of which some of the boundary is obscured in the image. These projects share the following drawbacks:

1. They may be easily hindered by noisy data and obscured boundaries (as is the case for the kidney in abdominal CAT scans);

---

*This type of knowledge was used by Liu et al. to extract bone shapes, although it is a much more elaborate and successful approach than thresholding [Liu, 1978].

2. They are semiautomatic, and a user must interactively suggest a starting point; and

3. The result is a bulky and unknowledgeable solution, i.e., the set of voxels that belong to an organ have no concise shape description.

The diagnostician, when analyzing CAT scans, utilizes quantitative, relational, and geometric types of knowledge. It is the anticipated shape of an organ and its expected locus that triggers his recognition. Some of the organs are easy to locate: the spinal column is one of them. Based on the location of distinguished organs, other organs, which are harder to locate, may then be discovered.

In this study, a new technique and theory for understanding 3-D images is developed, implemented, and tested. An associative network [Findler, 1979] is used to represent the knowledge for gross anatomy within the domain in which spatial relations between organs are represented. *Generalized-Cylinders* (GC's) [Agin, 1972] provide building blocks for a detailed geometrical model of individual objects (organs). In general, the model as a whole is an associative network which associates quantitative, predicative, and geometric data with hierarchically related elements. In addition, procedural knowledge—as expert-routines—is embedded in the model in key positions to make important strategical decisions at fitting time. Image understanding is accomplished in a top-down iterative process in which a model-instance is fitted to the data. The system provides efficiency by a hierarchical and parallel fitting process, as well as a pyramid-of-resolutions organization of the 3-D image data.

The contributions of this work pertain to the following important issues:

1. The extension of the geometric complexity of GC's by letting each cross section, as well as the main axis, be a free-form curve, with the use of cubic uniform B-spline curves. This extension GC is important compared to previous restrictive definitions (and use) of this tool (cf. Table 2.2 in Chapter 2).

2. The representation and utilization of relational geometrical knowledge of a 3-D domain for the purpose of understanding a 3-D image taken from it.

3. The development, implementation, and testing of a technique for the hierarchical 3-D fitting of objects to 3-D data.

4. The efficient handling of huge amounts of data in a 3-D image by a top-down, parallel approach, and a pyramid-of-resolution organization of the 3-D image data.

5. The development of display techniques for 3-D shapes.

6. A general approach, applicable to a large variety of useful areas where *a priori* knowledge about the scene is available, for which a specific model can be built and used for an automatic image analysis.

1.6 Long-Range Benefits

Before projecting the benefits of an automatic analysis of CAT scans, we will examine the current uses of CAT scans in medicine.

1. *Tumor discovery:* Tumors (cancers) are small pieces of abnormal tissue that are detected either by direct visualization of their image in a scan with the aid of contrast material (they usually have differing density from the surrounding healthy tissue), or by observation of changes in shape or location of surrounding organs.

2. *Treatment planning:* One of the more effective means of treating tumors is that in which the patient is irradiated in such a way that most of the radiation energy is absorbed by the abnormal tissue, which is thus destroyed by radiation damage to the replication mechanism of the cells. To minimize the damage to healthy tissue, the patient is radiated in collimated rays, from a large number of directions, so that the rays intersect at the location of the tumor. The design and calculation of the paths for these rays is aimed at maximizing the dose to the tumor while minimizing the dose to other tissues. CAT images are used for this purpose to reveal the inside anatomy of soft tissues as well as hard ones [Sunguroff, 1978].

   Another field in which an accurate view of the internal structure of an organ is desired in brain surgery, where tiny parts of brain tissue (or tumors) must be destroyed by means of inserted electrodes.

3. *Noninvasive vivisection:* The most intuitive use of CAT scans is for the purpose of having a more favorable view of a patient's anatomy. A surgeon can scan his patient before operating on him, to prevent any unpleasant "surprises" at the actual operation.

This study is an attempt to provide an intelligent tool for diagnostic medicine, and it follows the current trend of adding computer power to help daily medicine practices (an example of an on-going project in this respect is reported by Lemke [1979]). Computerized networks that include medical imaging devices like CAT and NMR scanners, called PACS (for Picture

Archiving and Communications Systems [Dwyer, 1983]), are fertile environments in which our system can be greatly beneficial. The successful automatic evaluation of CAT images will significantly enhance their usefulness and effectiveness as a diagnostic aid in the following ways:

1. *Automating the manual processing of CAT scans* as discussed in the first part of this section (tumor discovery, noninvasive vivisection, and treatment planning).

2. *Providing 3-D representation of organs* to overcome the 2-D barrier of current methods for viewing CAT scans (as slices and cross sections). Figure 1.4 illustrates the 3-D graphic display of organs that is produced by the system presented in this thesis.

3. *Scanning planning:* an integrated setup in which the scans are analyzed in real-time. The automatic analyzing system interacts with the scanner. A typical scenario is as follows. The physician requests a scan of a particular organ. The scanner is activated for a few sparse scans at low resolution (i.e., at low radiation doses and in short scanning time). The low-resolution image is analyzed, and a more accurate prediction as to the organ location is made. Further, denser scanning can then take place at a high resolution and at a more correct location. The final result is that the physician gets a scan of the desired location in the body in shorter time, with a smaller radiation dose to his patient (this may be compared to a manual examination of *SCOUT VIEW®* (see [Herman, 1980]).

4. *Surgical simulation* to introduce a new dimension in medicine for both educational and experimental purposes (although surgical simulation is still in the early stages of research). It is motivated largely by cases in which a surgeon has to repeat an operation, or by other occasions when several surgical techniques are available, so that the best one can be chosen. The provision of 3-D view of organs is very suitable for the phase of interaction with the surgeon in a simulation session before the actual operation takes place.

® Trademark of the General Electric Company.

2

Organ Modeling: Generalized-Cylinders

The rationale for the model-driven approach to understanding 3-D CAT images was explained in the introduction. Such an approach is common in 2-D image analysis, and it will be discussed further in Chapter 6. In this chapter, I shall present the arguments for and details of the geometric modeling of individual organs as Generalized-Cylinders. A higher level of modeling that will include knowledge of the gross anatomy (i.e., the interorgan spatial relations) will be explained in the next chapter.

2.1 Purpose

Organ modeling is used to represent the 3-D geometry of objects found in the human abdominal anatomy. In choosing a representation, such anatomical characteristics of the human domain as those that follow should be taken into account:

1. Most of the organs have longitudinal axes that mimic the organs' shapes, as illustrated in Figure 2.1.

2. Most organs are smooth (Figure 2.2).

The intuitive approach to this problem is to let the model be flexible enough to allow an initial geometry, represented parametrically, to be matched against the actual anatomy of the organ, and modified accordingly. The model-directed approach starts with a prototypical shape and changes it to fit individual data. For example, if we imagine that the kidney is initially modeled of clay in the shape of an egg, the fitting process will bend, distort, or scale the shape until it conforms to the actual kidney image data. To achieve this shape modification, we would like to have control of the location in space of individual points on its surface. In the work reported here, a parametric representation is used, since only few such points are needed, their number being dependent upon the geometric complexity of the shape.

Figure 2.1   By drawing the main axes that are typical to the
               various organs, one perceives the skeletal description
               of the human anatomy.

HEAD,

HANDS, SPINAL-
        COLUMN,

LIVER,

KIDNEYS,

HIPS,

LEGS.

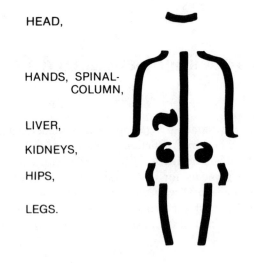

Figure 2.2   Most organs are smooth,as presented by these
               drawings of the kidney and liver.

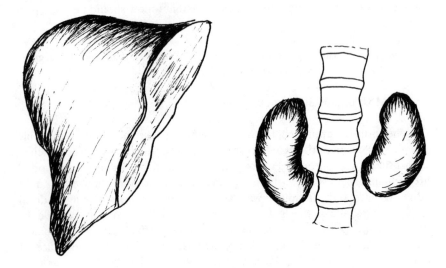

2.2 Possible 3-D Representations

Quite a few representations for 3-D geometric shapes are feasible, many of which were surveyed by Badler and Srihary ([Badler, 1978; Srihary, 1981]). Below are some of the parametric representations for the geometry of 3-D objects that were considered here.

Boxes and Cylinders—PADL. The PADL system [Voelcker, 1978] focuses on computer-aided design and manufacture of solid objects. Solid objects can be modeled and/or made by machines; the combination of solid parametric primitives such as boxes and cylinders permits a wide range of applications. However, since the PADL primitives are not smooth (the combination of cylinders and boxes leaves many sharp edges [see Figure 2.3]), the PADL system for the representation of solid objects was excluded from consideration for application in this research.

Figure 2.3   The PADL representation of solid objects as the combination of boxes and cylinders. Objects are made by adding and subtracting such volumes from each other. (Printed with permission of the PADL project at the University of Rochester, Rochester, N. Y., ©1979, all rights reserved.)

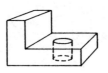

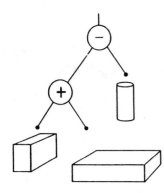

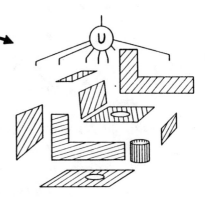

Spherical harmonics [Schudy, 1980]. The spherical harmonics technique is restricted to surfaces that can be defined as a function on a sphere. Spherical harmonics may be favored for applications where the modeled object is mostly isotropic, i.e., it does not have an obvious longitudinal axis. Figure 2.4 presents the analytic definition of a spherical harmonic surface and some examples. This representation is controlled by parameters, the number of which depends on the surface details needed: high-order coefficients yield higher surface spatial details. The model is flexible and (as shown by Schudy) is ideal for fitting and matching against 3-D images of surfaces which are mostly isotropic. A main drawback is the illocality of parameters, i.e., there is no way to relate a parameter to a specific point, or a limited locus, on the surface.

Figure 2.4   The analytic definition of the spherical-harmonics used by Schudy, and some examples of surfaces defined by them.

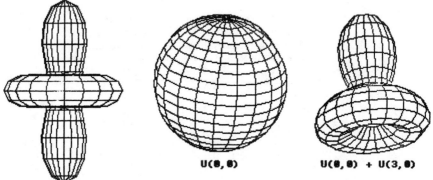

U(●, ●)   U(●, ●) + U(3, ●)

U(●, ●) + U(4, ●)

$$R(\Theta, \Phi) \quad = A_{0,0} + U_{0,0} +$$

$$\sum_{m=1}^{M} \sum_{n=0}^{m} \left(A_{m,n} U_{m,n}(\Theta, \Phi) + B_{m,n} V_{m,n}(\Theta, \Phi) \right)$$

where:

$$U_{m,n}(\Theta, \Phi) = \cos n\Theta \cdot \sin^n \Phi \cdot P_m^{(n)}(\cos \Phi)$$
$$for \; m = 0, \ldots, M; \; n = 0, \ldots, m;$$

$$V_{m,n}(\Theta, \Phi) = \sin n\Theta \cdot \sin^n \Phi \cdot P_m^{(n)}(\cos \Phi)$$
$$for \; m = 1, \ldots, M; \; n = 1, \ldots, m;$$

and:

$P_m^{(n)}$ **is the n-*th*   derivative of the m-*th*   Legendre polynomial.**

Generalized-Cylinders (GC) [Agin, 1972]. The Generalized-Cylinders technique was motivated by the need to represent objects such as organs and other living shapes. The original application was to represent a 3-D object that has a longitudinal axis and a smoothly changing cross section along that axis. Later uses of this technique were the modeling of animals and the automatic recognition of such shapes from 2-D images [Marr & Nishihara, 1977]. The use of a restricted class of GC's to model organs for the purpose of understanding 3-D images was first done by [Soroka, 1979]. GC's are ideal for modeling objects such as organs, since they are constructed around the typical longitudinal axis and they provide for a smooth surface.

Bivariate (tensor product) surfaces [Coons, 1967]. The bivariate surfaces technique is mainly used for CAD/CAM (Computer-Aided Design/Computer-Aided Manufacture) in which surfaces of arbitrary shapes and complexity are desired for the design of mechanical parts. In this representation, the convenience of manual manipulations and the efficiency of graphic display are major factors. Because this technique is very general, one must specify what univariate functions are used in the definition of the tensor products. Being a surface representation, it is not suited for representing an enclosed volume, such as we intend to represent in modeling an organ. Furthermore, similar surfaces can have distinctively different parametric representations, making comparisons difficult.

Polygons and triangulation [Gouraud, 1971; Fuchs, 1977; Brown, 1978]. In the polygons and triangulation method the surface is represented as a collection of planar polygons that are defined by the 3-D coordinates of their corners. A common representation for surfaces in this category is triangulation, in which the polygons are only triangles. The generalization to polygons is motivated by certain types of computer graphics in which the display of curved objects, with the full effect of hidden surface elimination, is desired. The representation of smooth, continuous surfaces by a technique which uses units that are not smooth themselves imposes a natural problem. This problem may be overcome by increasing the number of polygons while decreasing their sizes. Figure 2.5 presents the triangulation of a human face in a technique developed by Fuchs. The major disadvantage of triangulation for the purpose of this research is that, besides being basically a surface representation, the representation is nonparametric.

Spheres [Badler, 1977]. This technique uses a single-volume primitive, the sphere, and composes the object representation from the union of such spheres in varying sizes and at particular locations. In this technique, the shape is represented by a limited number of parameters, depending on the desired object description details (Figure 2.6).

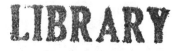

Figure 2.5   Triangulation of the human head. The triangulation is
based on a given set of contour polylines, and is
solved under the constraint that the defined surface
will have the minimal area of all possible
triangulations. (From "Optimal surface reconstruction
from planar contours," by H. Fuchs, Z.M. Kedem,
and S.P. Uselton. Commun. ACM 20 (10), October
©1977 by the Association for Computing Machinery,
Inc., all rights reserved.)

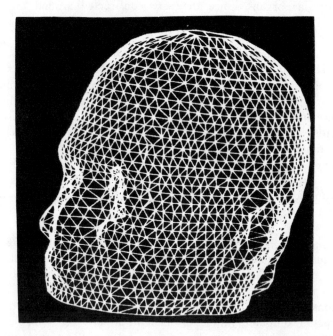

Oct-trees [Srihary, 1981; 1982]. The single volume primitives are parallelpipes, much like the voxels in 3-D images. There is a hierarchical structure imbedded in an oct-tree, which is a tree with a unified branching factor of 8. In essence, this is a generalization of *quad-trees* [Samet, 1982], it is data-oriented, volume-representation and is unfit for our application as is the spheres technique above.

All these possibilities are compared in Table 2.1 as to their usefulness for the representation of organ shape, their descriptive power, and their deficiencies.

2.3 Chosen Representation: Generalized-Cylinders (GC's)

A Generalized-Cylinder is built around the notion of a "main axis" and a smoothly changing cross section. It has favorable attributes for directing and

Figure 2.6   The representation of the human body as the volume
union of spheres. (From "A representation and
display system for the human body and other 3-D
curved objects," by N.I. Badler and J. O'Rourke,
Computer Science Department, University of
Pennsylvania, all rights reserved.)

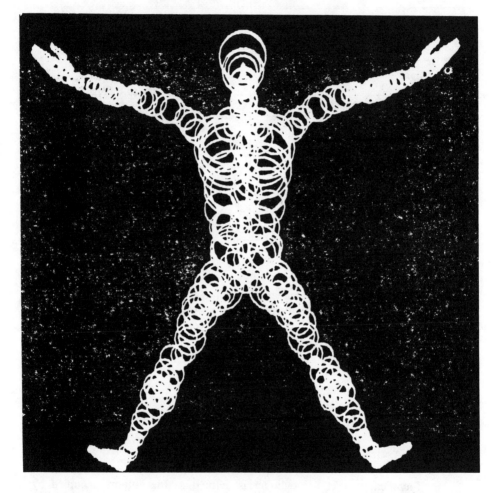

serving as a basis for the search and detection of 3-D objects in a 3-D image. We
shall survey uses of GC's in the past and provide a precise definition of a more
general GC and the mathematical tools for manipulating it.

2.3.1 Theory of Generalized-Cylinders

[Agin, 1972] used GC's to model primitive 3-D shapes as part of the *hand-eye*
robotics project at Stanford University. His purpose was to represent objects

Table 2.1.   A Comparison of Methods for Computer Representation of
3-D Objects with Respect to Their Usefulness, Deficiencies, and
Descriptive Power.

METHOD	ADVANTAGES	DISADVANTAGES	APPROPRIATE FOR REPRESENTING:
PADL	Simple, few primitives.	Sharp edges. Restricted curved surfaces.	Mechanical parts. Man-made objects. Basically, volume rep.
Spherical Harmonics	Shape controlled by hierarchy of parameters. Efficiently computable	Parameters are non-local.	Objects that are mostly isotropic, not long and curving. Surface representation.
Generalized-Cylinders	Hierarchical structure. Efficiently computable. Locally controlled.	Can be ambiguous, not everything is physically realizable.	Natural objects, smooth with typical longitude axis. Both volume and surface representation.
Tensor Product	Powerful parametric surface representation.	Hard to relate to volume of objects. Hard to match.	Any surface.
Polygons, Triangles	Powerful surface representation. Relatively simple.	Inefficient for curved objects. Nonparametric.	Polyhedra. Surface representation.
Spheres Oct-trees	Simple single primitive.	Nonsmooth surface. Nonparametric. Hard to match.	Volume representation.

that are scanned by a calibrated laser beam and a TV camera (the *Triangulation Laser System*). The scan result is a set of points on the object's surface, given, within some degree of accuracy, by their space location. The Generalized-Cylinder method, also known as the method of *Generalized Translational Invariance,* is defined as:

1.   A space curve, called the axis.

2.   Planes perpendicular to the axis, and a set of axes on the plane.

3.   A variable cross section described on these axes.

Technically, a classic cylinder is defined as the volume occupied by "sweeping" (translating) a disk perpendicular to a straight line—the axis— bound to some sweeping-rule. When the axis is allowed to be an arbitrary space curve and the disc is allowed to vary while being swept (translated), we get a Generalized-Cylinder. Although the GC is considered a volume representation, it can easily serve as a surface representation by considering a planar curve (frame) instead of a plate, and thinking of the surface area "swept" by that curve as the GC.

Formally, the main axis is a space curve $\vec{A}(s)$, where s is a parameter that varies from 0 to 1 along the curve. In terms of the Cartesian coordinate system:

$$\vec{A}(s) = [X_A(s), \ Y_A(s), \ Z_A(s)] \ 0 \le s \le 1 \tag{2.1}$$

where each $X_A(s)$, $Y_A(s)$, and $Z_A(s)$ is a univariate function of the parameter s. A planar curve $\vec{C}(t)$ on the X-Y plane is defined in a similar way:

$$\vec{C}(t) = [X_C(t), \ Y_C(t), \ 0] \ 0 \le t \le 1 \tag{2.2}$$

To serve as a cross section for a Generalized-Cylinder, this curve is closed, so that $\vec{C}(0) = \vec{C}(1)$. A point on the surface of the cylinder is, therefore, a bivariate function of s and t:

$$\vec{D}(s,t) = \vec{A}(s) + X_C(t) \cdot \vec{X}(s) + Y_C(t) \cdot \vec{Y}(s) \tag{2.3}$$

In this case, $\vec{X}(s)$ and $\vec{Y}(s)$ are space vectors that represent the directions of the plane axes in which the curve $\vec{C}(t)$ is defined. $\vec{Z}(s)$, which doesn't appear in Eq. 2.3, is a third vector that is orthogonal to $\vec{X}(s)$ and $\vec{Y}(s)$ and is also the tangent to the curve $\vec{A}(s)$ at the point where the cross section is calculated. $\vec{X}$, $\vec{Y}$, and $\vec{Z}$ represent the effect of a sweeping-rule by defining the *orientation* of a cross-section curve that was swept along the main axis from one endpoint ($s = 0$) to some other point ($s > 0$). A second variable, in addition to the orientation of the *plane* in which the curve is defined, is an additional angle Θ, which represents the amount of rotation applied to the curve within its plane. A third variation that may occur during the sweep is change in the curve's shape. In the original GC's ([Agin, 1972]), limited systematic changes like linear scaling, as a function of s, were applied. In our GC's, the cross-section shape is *interpolated* through a set of cross-section curves at discrete locations along the main axis.

To calculate $\vec{X}$, $\vec{Y}$, and $\vec{Z}$, given some in-plane rotation Θ, Agin used the curvature (K) and torsion (T) of the main axis curve in the following equations:

$$\frac{\partial}{\partial s} X = -KZ \, \cos\Theta + TY$$

$$\frac{\partial}{\partial s} Y = KZ \, \sin\Theta - TX \tag{2.4}$$

$$\frac{\partial}{\partial s} Z = K(X \, \cos\Theta + Y \, \sin\Theta)$$

At every point along the curve $\vec{A}(s)$, an integral solution to this set of differential equations is needed.

2.3.2 Previous Uses of Generalized-Cylinders

Agin. In Agin's work, simple shapes, mostly isolated, were automatically described as a collection of primitive GC's. These primitives were combined in a hierarchical structure via "joints." There were simple "end-to-end" joints and more complicated "t-joints." Although no satisfactory solution was given to the joints problem, this system performed fairly well in providing a segmentation of slit-scanned objects (e.g., a doll) into such primitives (cf. Figure 2.7). The primitive GC's used by Agin had circular cross sections, and the main axis curve was some analytic function (e.g., a polynomial).

Figure 2.7   A description of a doll as a collection of Generalized-Cylinders of circular cross section and analytically defined main axis (snake shapes). (From "Computer Description of Curved Objects" by G.J. Agin and T.O. Binford, *IEEE Transactions on Computers*, C-25, April 1976, © 1976 by IEEE Inc., all rights reserved.)

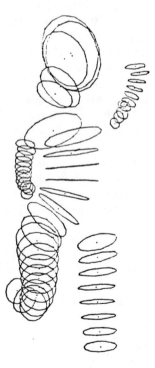

Nevatia & Binford. The GC's idea was extended further by [Nevatia & Binford, 1977], who based their work also on the triangulation laser system for scanning 3-D scenes. The purpose of this work was not only to represent such objects but to *recognize* them as well. For that purpose they needed to segment the objects properly and used the definition of GC's for the correct (and unambiguous) selection of main axes for the various primitive parts of the shapes. Once such axes were found, they provided a stick representation of the shape. This description was matched against a stored visual data-base of possible objects, to result in a scene interpretation. GC's in this work were defined in this very general way: arbitrary cross sections perpendicular to an arbitrary space curve. The approach was "bottom-up" and consisted in the extrapolation of GC's based on some previously discovered cross sections. Cross sections were defined as the planar polygons generated by intersecting the surface data points with a plane. The constraints that the main axis be normal to the plane and that it pass through the "center of gravity" of the cross section and not intersect with other cross sections guided its selection. In general, the main axis was a space polyline, while the cross sections were polygons. This was sufficient, since no surface details were required, merely a volume representation. In fact, the internal representation of the GC's did not rely at all on surface details but emphasized other GC characteristics, such as the two end-points, for the purpose of resolving "joints" problems. The internal representation for GC's included seven measurements:

1. Length of axis

2. Average width of cross sections

3. Average width of cross sections at both endpoints

4. Length to width ratio

5. Average cone angle (some characteristics of the GC)

6. Axis direction and position at each endpoint

7. The polygons at each endpoint.

Marr & Nishihara. [Marr & Nishihara, 1976] used the GC for a purpose similar to that of Nevatia but on a different type of data: 2-D images. GC's served to represent 3-D objects (animals) in a hierarchical structure of a "stick figure." This was a volume segmentation of the complex shapes in scenes, and GC's were represented by their main axis (straight line) and their width (diameter of circular cross sections). This hierarchical representation could go into any level of detail in a recursive manner with the intention to compare it to a set of templates from a data-base, to result in a symbolic interpretation of the scene.

Soroka.   Yet another use of the GC, for a purpose similar to the purpose of this work, is reported in [Soroka, 1979; 1981]. Soroka used GC's in a very restrictive way (he called them "Generalized Cones"), requiring that all cross sections be parallel conics perpendicular to the main axis, which is a straight line. These restrictions are due partially to the fact that the data, 3-D CAT images, were perceived as a set of 2-D images, or slices. Soroka's approach was mainly bottom-up, though it also involved some top-down processes, and was aimed at recognizing the objects in the scene (organs) by representing them as some combination of Generalized Cones.

Table 2.2 presents a comparison of the various uses of GC's to the particular way that they are used in this thesis.

Table 2.2.   Comparison of the Uses of Generalized-Cylinders in
the Previous Works by Agin, Nevatia, Marr & Nishihara,
Soroka and Shani

RESEARCHER	SCENE and IMAGE	BUILDING BLOCKS	PURPOSE/ REPRESENTATION
Agin	Isolated simple shapes with longitudinal axis. 3-Dimensional images.	*Main axis:* analytic function *Cross sections:* circles. Main axis pass through approx. centroid, perpendicular to cross sections.	Parametric representation of objects in the scene. Volume representation.
Nevatia	Complex scenes of compound objects. 3-Dimensional images.	*Main axis:* polyline. *Cross sections:* polygons in arbitrary orientations. Main axis pass through centroids and perpendicular to cross sections.	Recognition of Objects. Scene interpretation.
Marr	2-dimensional pictures of animals.	*Main axis:* straight line. *Cross section:* circles. A volume skeleton made of simple cylinders.	Recognition of Objects. Scene interpretation.
Soroka	Parallel slices of 3-dimensional image. CAT scans.	*Main axis:* aribtrary curve. *Cross sections:* cone sections, parallel. Main axis pass through center of parallel cross sections.	Recovery of objects (organs) shape.
Shani	3-Dimensional image of the human abdomen. CAT scans.	*Main axis:* arbitrary B-spline *Cross sections:* arbitrarily oriented, arbitrary planar B-splines. Main axis pass through centroids, and perpendicular to cross sections.	Recognition and recovery of objects (organs) shape, scene interpretation.

Historically, the 2-D analogy of GC's as a representation of 2-D shapes was compared to *Medial Axis Transformation* [Blum, 1964] (also known as the method of "the prairie fire transformation"). Both methods come out with some skeletal transformation of the shape. GC's are, however, less vulnerable to small discontinuities in shape boundary.

The 2-D analogy to GC's was also pursued for solving the find-path problem in Robotics [Brooks, 1982]. Like Soroka, Brooks termed his primitives generalized cones. He used them to define the free space around obstacles that a robot has to move around.

The number of objects representable by GC's is certainly large; however, there are some situations for which a GC is mathematically, but not physically, feasible (Figure 2.8A). Other conflict occurs if we require that the main axis be both normal to the cross sections and pass through their centroid (Figure 2.8B). In such cases, we would prefer the orthogonality constraint, since it couples the orientation of cross sections and the shape of the main axis.

The benefits of having the main axis pass through the center of gravity (or centroid) of cross sections lie in the effective calculation of GC volume [Porter, 1962]. The volume of a GC is calculated by integrating the cross-sectional area along the curve. If Area(s) is the area of the cross section at point s on the main axis, then

$$Volume(GC) = \int_0^1 \left[Area(s) \times \frac{\partial}{\partial s} \, Length\left[\vec{A}(s)\right]\right] ds \qquad (2.5)$$

Figure 2.8   Some Generalized-Cylinders are physically impossible; A) The cross sections intersect each other; and B) The main axis may either pass through the center of cross sections or be perpendicular to them.

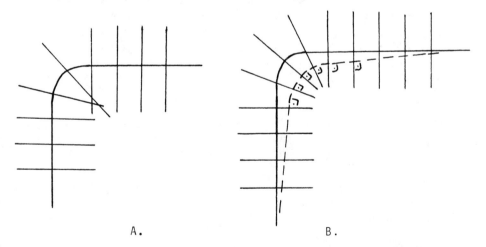

A.   B.

When the surface area of the GC is desired, then the main axis must go through the center of gravity of the frame curve of the cross sections (as opposed to the center of gravity of the solid plane enclosed in the cross section). A similar formula then works for the surface area.

2.3.3 Representation of GC's

In this work, GC's are defined in a way similar to the definition of Agin and Nevatia:

1. The main axis is a free-form continuous 3-D curve.

2. Each cross section is a closed free-form continuous plane curve.

3. Cross sections are perpendicular to the main axis.

4. The main axis passes through centroids of cross sections (or some approximation of them).

   (NOTE: There is no sweeping rule for cross sections, but they are interpolated through a discrete set of cross-section curves.)

Internally, GC's are represented as a *list* of cross sections. Each cross section is a closed, continuous curve, represented by a list of 2-D points along its periphery, also called *control points,* and a cross-section curve is interpolated through them. The points defining the cross section are given relative to the cross section's own coordinate system, which is assumed to be its center, i.e., location [0,0] is the centroid of the cross section. Each such *center point* is associated with a 3-D coordinate in the reference system for the GC itself. The main axis is a space curve that is interpolated through this list of 3-D points. In response, the main axis defines a normal vector in each such center point, which is used to calculate the orientations of the cross sections. Formally, a GC is defined as follows:

$< GC > ::= \{< \text{cross section} >_1, \ldots, < \text{cross section} >_N\}$

$< \text{cross section} > ::= (< \text{center point} >, < \text{control points} >)$

$< \text{center point} > ::= [X, Y, Z]$

$< \text{control points} > ::= \{< \text{knot} >_1, \ldots, < \text{knot} >_M\}$

$< \text{knot} > ::= [x, y]$

where: { ... }   denotes a list of items,
        ( )   denotes a pair of items, and
        [ ]   denotes a 2-D (or 3-D) coordinate.

In previous uses for GC's, cross sections and main-axis curves were polylines (Nevatia; Marr), polynomials (Agin), or close conics (Soroka); in this work curves are piece-wise polynomials, or more precisely, *splines.* An extensive discussion of *cubic uniform B-splines* is given in Appendix B. Cubic uniform B-splines are an efficient and popular means for interpolation of smooth curves through a set of *knot* points by cubic polynomial pieces. The theory of B-splines as developed by [DeBoor, 1979] and presented to CAD/CAM by [Riesenfeld, 1973] provides the following characteristics (when curves have parametric representation).

1.   Efficient interpolation. Every segment of the curve (a *span*) that goes between two knot points is easily interpolated by a set of matrix multiplications, most of which can be done once, ahead of time [Wu, 1977].

2.   Locality. The shape of each span is controlled only by the closest four knot points, so that changing one such a point will not affect the curve globally (as it will do with polynomials or cone sections, for example).

3.   Smoothness, with three degrees of continuity across knot points. Although each span is of a low degree (cubic), the points where spans meet enjoy continuity of displacement, slope, and curvature (for each of the parametric components).

4.   Affine transformable. Given a set of knot points, they define a curve. To find the affine transform of such a curve, all that is needed is to find the affine transform of the set of knot points. The curve defined by the transformed knot points is the desired one.

Several possibilities other than cubic B-splines for representing curves in the GC's definition were mentioned in the course of the above discussion. These possibilities and some others are summarized in Table 2.3.

Both the individual cross sections and the main axis are interpolated by the same means: uniform cubic B-splines. While cross-sectional curves are parameterized in X and Y, the main axis is parameterized in X, Y, and Z. The shape of the main axis is defined by the locations of the center points of individual cross sections. The shape of the main axis curve defines the orientation of planar cross-section curves. The details of how such an orientation is calculated are given in Appendix F. This situation is schematized in Figure 2.9: based on the tangent vectors and the locations of center points, an affine transformation is defined as a 4x4 matrix [Newman, 1976] which translates the 2-D definition of a cross section into a 3-D planar curve. In practice, all orientations are calculated by a special routine that returns a list of transformation matrices.

Table 2.3. A Comparison of Methods for Representing Cross-sections:
Polylines, Overhauser, Cone-sections, Polynomials, and B-splines.

METHOD	LOCALITY	# OF CONTROL POINTS FOR SMOOTH SURFACE	ACCURACY/ EFFICIENCY	SMOOTH	NOTES
Polygons	Yes	Many	High/High	No	Linear piecewise
Polynomials	No	Moderate	Low/Low	Yes	
Parabolic blending [Overhauser, 1968]	Yes	Moderate	Good/High	Yes	General free-form curves. Piecewise polynomials.
Cone-sections	No	Few	Good/Low	Yes	Restricted. Nongeneral
B-splines	Yes	Moderate	Good/High	Yes	Free-form curves. Piecewise polynomials.

Figure 2.9   A particular cross section of the Generalized-Cylinder is a planar parametric curve, $\vec{C}_{s_0}(t)$, that corresponds to point $\vec{A}[s_0]$ on the main axis. It is defined as $\vec{C}_{s_0}(t) = [X_{s_0}(t), Y_{s_0}(t)\ 0, 1]$, in its local coordinate system, where the parameter t ranges between 0 and 1. A) The transformation converts the normalized coordinate $[x,y,0,1]$ on the cross section to normalized coordinate $[x',y',z',1]$ in the cylinder's 3-D coordinate system. The point $[x',y',z',1]$ is located on a plane perpendicular to the tangent to the main axis at point $A(s)$. Relative to the system $(\vec{X}', \vec{Y}')$ on this plane, the curve is still $\vec{C}_s(t)$. The local axes $\vec{X}'$ and $\vec{Y}'$ are a function of the main-axis parameter s. B) The Frenet trihedron is defined by the three axes $\vec{A}(s)$, $\vec{T}(s)$ and $\vec{K}(s)$ which are the tangent, torsion and curvature, respectively, of the curve. We may define the local cross-section plane axes $\vec{X}'$ and $\vec{Y}'$ as the $\vec{K}$ and $\vec{T}$ axes.

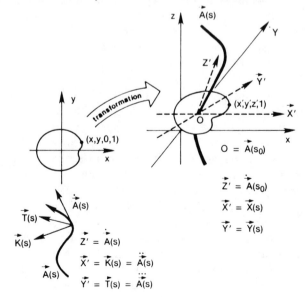

2.3.4 Helix Example

To demonstrate the power and correctness of this tool, a GC is defined for a helix made of circular cross sections with a "bump." Each cross-section curve of the helix is defined by six knot points. The example consists of two parts: a listing of the internal representation of the helix as a set of cross sections with center locations, and a graphic display of the helix surface by a wire-frame technique with hidden points eliminated (Figure 2.10 A,B).

Figure 2.10   Using the Generalized-Cylinder as a tool to represent a helix. A) The main axis and cross-section plane axis of the helix; B) The surface displayed as wire frame with hidden points eliminated.

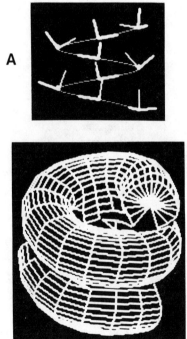

Part 1: The helix consists of nine cross sections. Each has a spline definition (that, in this case, are all the same and are shown only for the first two cross sections) and a center point:

→HELIX1

_____

Z Spline center: -30.0
Y Spline center: .000

X Spline center: 40.0
Spline values: real array [1:4,1:2]
[20.0] [.000]
[.000] [-20.0]
[-20.0] [10.0]
[.000] [20.0]

→HELIX2

Z Spline center: -20.0
Y Spline center: -40.0
X Spline center: .000
Spline values: real array [1:4,1:2]
[-20.0] [10.0]
[.000] [20.0]

→HELIX3	→HELIX4
Z Spline center: -10.0	Z Spline center: .000
Y Spline center: .000	Y Spline center: 40.0
X Spline center: -40.0	X Spline center: .000

→HELIX5	→HELIX6
Z Spline center: 10.0	Z Spline center: 20.0
Y Spline center: .000	Y Spline center: -40.0
X Spline center: 40.0	X Spline center: .000

→HELIX7	→HELIX8
Z Spline center: 30.0	Z Spline center: 40.0
Y Spline center: .000	Y Spline center: 40.0
X Spline center: -40.0	X Spline center: .000

→HELIX9

Z Spline center: 50.0
Y Spline center: .000
X Spline center: 40.0

Part 2: See Figure 2.10.

2.3.5 Summary

Cross sections of GC's are 2-D parametric curves that are defined as planar closed uniform cubic B-spline curves that interpolate through a set of knot points. The main axis is a 3-D parametric *open* uniform cubic B-spline curve that interpolates through the list of center-point locations of the individual cross sections. Depending on the shape of the main axis, orientations for the cross sections are defined as affine transformations that translate and orient each cross section from its 2-D definition (on the X-Y plane) to its position on the GC (Figure 2.9). These transformations are 4×4 matrices. The GC representation is parametric in the sense that few geometric values precisely define its shape. These parameters are local in that they control the GC shape in the close vicinity of their space location. As demonstrated in the helix example above, it is a very powerful means of describing 3-D shapes for graphics display. The power of this tool for modeling will be presented in the ensuing chapters.

In an attempt to establish a rigorous mathematical foundation for GC's, Shafer and Kanade [1983] developed and proposed a system for categorizing the various GC's. They introduced an additional degree of freedom into the definition of GC's as the angle of inclination, α, which is the angle between the main axis and a cross section. In Soroka's case this was fixed, but differs from $\pi/2$. In our case it is fixed at $\pi/2$, but the arbitrary shape of main-axis curve allows cross-sections not to be parallel to each other. In Shafer's terminology, our GC's are categorized as RGC (for Right Generalized Cylinders).

3

Fitting Strategy and Model Structure

3.1 Introduction

This chapter is concerned with the central computational paradigms that underlie the fitting strategy which is integrated into a hierarchical model. In fitting, a model is matched against image data and updated accordingly. The focus is a goal-oriented approach: an image is not analyzed "blindly" but with the purpose of finding some features which measure its deviation from a model.

Fitting a model for an arbitrarily complicated 3-D shape may pose some difficult problems. Following a well-practiced technique from artificial intelligence (AI), we *decompose* the shape-fitting problem into simpler problems, for which fitting may be easier.

Modeling organs by Generalized-Cylinders leads to a natural decomposition of 3-D shapes into simpler elements of decreased dimensionality. We will define such decomposition as *shape-refinement* to contrast it with other common techniques in which decomposed elements are of similar dimensionality to the original one. It is convenient to refer to these other techniques as *primitivization,* since the term corresponds to its traditional use in AI.

In the first part of this chapter, differences between these two methods and their relation to a goal-oriented approach will be discussed, revealing also the hierarchies of our model. Next, the model geometry is presented, level by level. The fundamental computational paradigms follow. These paradigms define principles for a successive subdivision of a goal to subgoals and then define ways to combine solutions to subgoals into one solution to a goal, and so forth. It turns out that goal/subgoal relations fit very well into the "shape-refinement" of a GC. A substantial use of knowledge guides the creation of goals and subgoals in the fitting process. This knowledge, largely geometric, is organized hierarchically by the model levels, as an associative network. Implementation details are deferred to the next chapter.

3.2 Primitivization and Shape Refinement

Traditionally, primitivization works by decomposing a model for a complicated shape into a collection of simple, tractable components (primitives) and providing tools and rules to combine them into the original model. There are several reasons for this approach:

1. Relatively few parameterized shape primitives can yield a large class of shapes.

2. Simple primitive objects present simple, tractable versions of the general problem, for each of which a complete solution can be found (as a function of some parameters).

3. Few combining rules solve some high-level problems based on abstract notions presented by the primitives, on the condition that there are a very small number of primitives.

Some examples of such approaches are 1) PADL (primitives are boxes and cylinders); 2) Badler's spheres (one primitive, a sphere); and 3) Rubin's boxes (a single primitive, a box that is used to model complex scenes for the purpose of their rapid graphic rendering [Rubin, 1980]), or the oct-tree representation; and more.

Our differing approach is to *shape-refine* a model. The elements of such decomposition are not just simplified versions of the general case (with the same dimensionality) but, rather, have reduced geometric space dimensionality. One would include in this category the various skeleton representations where the skeleton of a 3-D solid object is an entirely different entity, with different dimensionality, but one which would serve well as a representation of the important model characteristics for a given problem (cf. [Blum, 1964; Marr & Nishihara, 1976]). Modeling an object as a collection of surfaces is a similar approach, since a 3-D shape is made from a combination of 2-D elements.

Generalized-Cylinders for modeling organs are better suited to the shape-refinement approach than to primitivization. This was not always the case in previous uses of GC's (cf. 2.3.2). Soroka used Generalized Cones, as variants of a primitive GC, which were combined volumetrically to produce more general shapes of organs. Nevatia & Binford, and Agin, have used GC's as the (relatively complex) primitive of a shape model and combined them via "joints" at their end points. GC's are both volume and surface representations, having no natural simple primitive element (although one may think of a classic cylinder as such a primitive, he will find it difficult to define Generalized-Cylinders in terms of combining solid classic cylinders). In this work, organs are modeled by Generalized-Cylinders whose definition (cf. 2.3.3 above) reveals a hierarchy of elements with a gradually changing geometric complexity:

- The organ is a 3-D volume enclosed by a smooth surface that has a longitudinal axis. It is referred to as the *organ-level.*

- An organ is composed of 2-D cross sections, each of which is a planar area enclosed by a smooth curve, and which are considered in the *cross-section level.*

- The curve of a cross section is itself a 1-D entity, elements of which are in the *boundary-point level.*

To complete the hierarchical structure, there is the

- *Top-level,* which deals with multiple 3-D objects in a 3-D environment. This level is also referred to here as the *gross anatomy.*

Elements in the various model levels have only father-son relations, i.e., the only dependencies are of an element and its direct descendants. There are no communications between "brother" elements, as depicted in Figure 3.1.

Figure 3.1   Components of the hierarchical model have strictly tree relations of a node and its immediate descendants, and vice versa. There are three types of relations: 1) search invocation, 2) results propagation, and 3) modificitons. These relations correspond to the three fitting phases in Section 3.4.

CONTROL STRUCTURE :

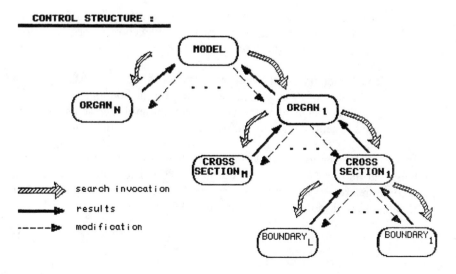

This tree relation is important for both 1) potential parallelism in applying model elements in a matching process, and 2) utilization of the basic goal/subgoal computational paradigm, whose components are presented in Figure 3.1 as three control relations between tree elements.

3.3 Geometry: Hierarchical Coordinate Systems

In the model, there are four types of coordinate systems that correspond to the four model levels with the appropriate dimensions. There are also convenient and efficient geometric interfaces between systems of related elements (cf. Figure 3.1) that can transform a point in a coordinate system of one model element to a corresponding point in the system for its father element. The coordinate systems are depicted in Figure 3.2, and are defined as follows:

1. The body coordinate system corresponds to the top level of multiple 3-D objects (GC's). This system references the image data and is a 3-D right-hand Cartesian system, where Z goes upward, X goes from left to right, and Y goes forward. The body is located in the first and fifth space octants thus defined. The X-Y plane intersects the body at roughly the *xiphisternal joint*, a situation which is expected to be accomplished manually during CAT scanning by the scanner technicians.

2. The organ coordinate system is a 3-D Cartesian system, centered on the Generalized-Cylinder that defines the organ (object), so that the longitudinal axis goes approximately along the Z axis, and the cross sections are approximately parallel to the X-Y plane.

3. The coordinate system for a cross section is 2-D only, and is centered on the corresponding closed curve, in its centroid, or some close approximation to the centroid.

4. The boundary-point coordinate system is 1-D and has its origin (location 0 of its single axis) at a point on the boundary of an organ model. An element in the boundary-point level represents a straight line segment, coplanar and normal to a cross-section curve.

An interface between two coordinate systems is an affine transformation, represented as a 4 × 4 matrix [Newman, 1975]. Each coordinate system essentially references a manifold or a subspace of a higher level space. For example, if x_b is a point in a 1-D boundary-level system, then

$$[x_c, \ y_c, \ 0, \ 1] = [x_b, \ 0, \ 0, \ 1] \cdot T_b \qquad (3.1)$$

Figure 3.2   Four coordinate systems for each of the four model
              levels. Each is originated at the geometric center of
              the corresponding model element. Affine
              transformations will translate the coordinate of a
              location in one system to the corresponding one in its
              predecessor element.

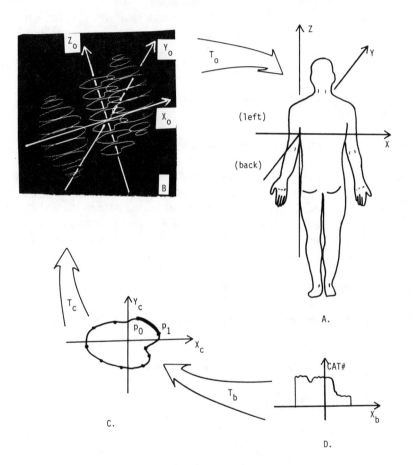

where $[x_c, y_c]$ is the coordinate of the point in the corresponding 2-D cross-section coordinate system.

The other transformation matrices play similar roles; a T_c matrix interfaces between a cross section and an organ, and a T_o transforms between an organ and the body. These transformations are either stored in the model or recalculated occasionally. Finally, to relate a point in a boundary-level element to the image data, we concatenate all the transformations that are defined along the path from the boundary-level element to the top level (cf. Figure 3.1):

$$[x, y, z, 1] = [x_b, 0, 0, 1] \cdot T_b \cdot T_c \cdot T_o \qquad (3.2)$$

Here, $[x, y, z]$ is the coordinate in the image that corresponds to x_b on one of the boundary-point-level elements.

3.4 Basic Hierarchical Matching Paradigms

In this work, in order to achieve a solution to the problem of understanding a 3-D image, we create a model-instance that consists only of the geometric attributes of the model, match this model-instance against the data, and modify it accordingly. The process, controlled by the *a priori* knowledge contained in the model itself, makes intensive use of heuristics; such heuristics are hereafter referred to as *basic computational paradigms*.

3.4.1 Hierarchical Problems

Each model element, at every level, has a set of distinctive four components to be considered in the fitting process:

- The corresponding element of the *model-instance.*

- The corresponding element of the *model* itself.

- The corresponding (sub) *image.*

- The corresponding *problem.*

The *model-instance* and the *model* components are the corresponding elements of the model and its instance, and represent geometric shape definitions and knowledge. The image component is a subimage that directly relates to the coordinate system defined at the appropriate model element. For elements at the various levels, the image component breaks down as follows:

- For the *top-level* it is the whole image data.

- For the *organ-level* it is a 3-D window (box) cut out of the image data and centered around the expected location of the organ.

- For the *cross-section level* it is the planar cross section of the image (at an arbitrary orientation, so that it should not be confused with the parallel data slices) centered around the expected centroid of a particular cross section of a GC.

- For the *boundary-point level* it is a 1-D subimage, made of the data values along a coplanar line segment (on the cross-section plane) normal to a cross-section curve, centered around the point where a boundary (i.e., change in image values) is expected.

The *problem* component at each level consists of matching a model-instance and an image relative to the same coordinate system, evaluating their difference, and suggesting a modification in the shape of the instance to compensate for that difference. The matching is based upon the notion of boundaries: that of the searched object and that of the model-instance. For example, at the organ level, the boundary is a 2-D surface of a 3-D object. Parametrically, $S(s,t) = [x,y,z]$ is the set of points on that surface as a function of the two surface parameters s and t. If we draw a normal to the model instance surface at some point $[s,t]$ and find that the object surface (boundary) is encountered at distance $D(s,t)$, then

$$M = \int\int |D(s,t)|\, ds\ dt \qquad (3.3)$$

is some measure for how good a match we have. The value of M can be interpreted as the volume difference between the searched object and the model instance. The pictorial interpretation of M, and its counterparts at the three lower levels, are depicted in Figure 3.3. Evidently, the problems at the cross-section level and the boundary-point levels are of gradually reduced dimensionality. The problem for a boundary-point element is completely trivial, being a problem in 1-D vision! At each of the levels, one may solve the problem by a least-square fitting of the model to the data. The approach taken here is different, since it takes into account the fact that the data may be noisy, have obscured boundaries, and unreliable boundary detectability. Clearly, if one can expect relatively distinguishable boundaries, one can try least-square fitting at each of the model elements to suggest a shape modification.

Figure 3.3   Decomposition of the fitting problem to components
of decreasing geometric dimensionality.

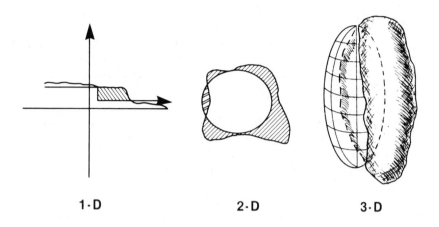

1·D   **2·D**   **3·D**

3.4.2 Basic Matching Paradigms

The problem confronting a model element at every level is to match a particular
model instance and a corresponding image; in other words, it is given a *goal*.
The fitting process iterates between matching and modification phases, and can
be done in one of two ways:

1. Each model element is presented with a goal, and iterates until
    reaching it.

2. The iteration is extended to the whole model tree and each element
    does only one step toward achieving its goal before confronting a new
    one, which is provided by a higher level element.

The first scheme eliminates any interference between the various model
levels and their elements, creating an unstructured process and avoiding any
benefit of the hierarchical model structure. Essentially, the only interesting
component in this case is the top level, which is supposed to solve the whole
problem without getting any help from the other components. Instead, we use
the second method of extending the iteration to the whole tree, executing a
complete tree traversal at each iteration, and repeating it until all problems and
subproblems have converged. Each iteration is accomplished in three phases
(these phases correspond to three types of arrows in Figure 3.1):

1. Defining the goal (problem) for each element;

2. Performing one step toward achieving that goal; and

3. Modifying the instance.

Phase 1 is a top-down operation of dividing a goal into subgoals. The goal presented to the top level is to find objects in a 3-D image, and all its descendants will be presented with some appropriate subgoals. Subgoals are then partially solved in phase 2, in low levels first and higher levels last, which is a bottom-up operation. The underlying principle for these two phases is further described as the *first basic computational paradigm*. Phase 3 is also a top-down process, underlined by the *second basic computational paradigm*.

3.4.3 The Goal/Subgoal Paradigm

Given an element in the model, it is confronted with a problem to solve that is within its capacity and limited to its geometrical complexity and dimension. If that component has descendants, instead of solving its problem by itself, it will break the problem into several subproblems so that each will fit into the capacity of these descendants, thus providing them with goals to achieve. These goals are considered a set of subgoals of the original goal, but they are simpler. Achievement of these goals will give a set of solutions to some simpler problems that can be combined and thus processed to solve the original, more complicated, one.

First Computational Paradigm:

Given a problem of a certain extent and complexity, it can be broken into *several* simpler problems, the solutions of which can be combined in order to solve the original, harder, problem.

This paradigm is interpreted at each level as follows:

1. *Top level.* In matching the model to data, try to find each organ separately; judge solutions to organ-finding problems based on gross-anatomy knowledge that consists of relational information.

2. *Organ level.* The 3-D organ model is a Generalized-Cylinder and will present each of its cross sections with a 2-D cross section of the image given to it. Each cross section will solve only a 2-D problem, which collectively will provide a solution to the 3-D problem confronted by this component.

3. *Cross-section level.* The 2-D cross-section model will present each of its descendants with a 1-D matching problem of searching in the vicinity of its boundary, normal to its outlining curve. Each solution returned by these components is 1-D in nature, but combined, they provide a 2-D solution.

4. *Boundary level.* Elements in this level have no descendants; they are very simple and trivial.

3.4.4 The Shape-modification Paradigm

Second Basic Computational Paradigm:

In modifying the model to make it fit better to the data, first apply the most global of such changes and add finest shape improvements last. By the same token, try simpler changes first; defer more complicated changes to a later stage.

Intuitively, one would not add the finest details to a sculpture before first applying coarse features—for example, one would outline first the general shape of a head before positioning eyes and other face details. The fitting of a 3-D shape to image data is analogous (cf. 2.1). Here 3-D changes dominate 2-D changes, which in turn dominate 1-D changes. The other aspect of this paradigm applies in making a decision about what to do first when a variety of options exist for modifications at the same level of detail (i.e., of the same dimensionality). Here, one would try gross changes first and, when those changes had been made, proceed to more detailed changes.

3.4.5 Heuristics and Experts

In essence, these paradigms are heuristics justified by intuition and common sense. There are, however, more concrete reasons for using them which evolve from the difficulties of analyzing 3-D images in the medical domain. Take, for example, the kidney in Figure 3.4; this is a 2-D cross section of an abdominal 3-D CAT scan. Note that the top-right boundary is obscured and only a portion of the kidney is clearly outlined. In Figure 3.4, a circular model is imposed on the image; it does not fit exactly, and a set of points outlines the supposedly correct kidney boundary as found by applying some local operators for edge detection on the image. Not all of them are good, and some are even misleading. It is clear that the right way is *not* to pick up the new set of points as the new boundary but to consider *all* the points as a *suggestion* for how to *change* the circle so that it will fit better with the image. Changes to the model (circle) can be done by:

- Translating it as a solid.

- Scaling it while preserving its shape.

- Distorting its shape, and so forth.

Figure 3.4   When fitting a cross section, the boundary of the
searched feature (the kidney boundary in this case) is
examined in the vicinity of the boundary suggested by
the model. A better boundary approximation is not
the collection of new points but a carefully modified
version of the model boundary that is guided by that
collection of points.

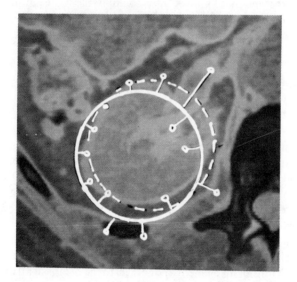

In other words, try to see how much can be done with the boundary as a *cross-sectional curve* before making an arbitrary change to it as a *collection of boundary points,* which is exactly what the second paradigm says.

A similar rationale is present in the relation between cross sections and a complete 3-D object. Here we try to see how much can be achieved in modifying a 3-D shape as a:

- Solid object.

- Solid shape.

- Flexible shape.

and only then as a *collection of cross sections.* The collection of points suggested in Figure 3.4 could be much more ill-positioned, had the appropriate image operators not been applied in the vicinity of the circle (under the assumption that it approximates the correct shape of the kidney cross section). The guided application of such operators is the essence of the first paradigm, and it is an important precondition for the useful application of the second paradigm. Another aspect of the difficulties in the fitting process is apparent if one examines Figure 3.4: it is the changing nature of object boundary for different organs and even for the same organ. To cope with that aspect, information about special cases of boundaries per organ (not per individual data) is encoded in procedures that are attached to model elements. These procedures are called *experts,* and there is one such expert per model element. An expert is the one that "knows" how to apply the basic paradigms during a fitting iteration. Not every element must have a unique expert; the variety needed depends on the variety and inhomogeneity of objects and difficulties that are expected in locating them.

3.5 Hierarchical Model Organization

3.5.1 Attributes Associations

Each element in each of the model levels is associated with some attributes. There are attributes of five different types: geometric, predicate, quantitative, strategic, and structural. The geometric attributes contain both the geometry of an element in reference to its own coordinate system and the interface between it and the levels above and below. The predicate attributes (for which the values are YES or NO) contribute to interorgan relations. The organ measurements of typical organ tissues are represented by the quantitative attributes. Strategy is mainly associated with expert routines, and structural attributes are the links between the details of an element at one level to the details of all its descendants at the next level.

Geometric mean and tolerance. In declaring geometrical attributes of the model, one cannot state firmly values like the size of an organ or its location, for the obvious reason that human bodies, though very much alike, differ and vary within some limits. For example, the spinal column is never at the front of the body but, within some tolerance of a normal position, at the back. The geometric attributes must, therefore, be some random variable. To simplify things we choose uniformly distributed random variables over a limited range for the geometric properties of the model. This distribution can be represented by a *mean value* and a *tolerance.* When an instance is modified, no one of its geometric attributes will be allowed to diverge from the given mean value by more than the given tolerance. Additional constraints are derived from the relation between brother elements as imposed by their common father element. The top level uses gross anatomy to constrain locations of "unreliable" organs (e.g., the kidney) by those of more robust organs (e.g., the spinal column), while the GC definition of the organ imposes constraints on the relative position of its cross sections (cf. Appendix F.2).

Figure 3.5   Associative network for gross-anatomy representation in the top level. The big dots represent organ nodes, and links are named *NEIGHBORHOOD$_i$*. Only some of the possible attributes are drawn.

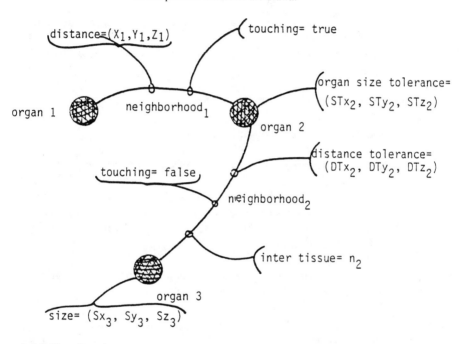

3.5.2 Top Level

The top level models the gross anatomy. Here, model geometric primitives are combined in an associative network [Brachman, 1979]. Figure 3.5 represents such a network. This structure will be discussed and explained further in the next chapter. Pairs of organs are linked, and various attributes are attached to those links. These attributes are based on statistical studies and on *a priori* knowledge of the scanning procedure. For instance, the patient is laid upon his back on the supporting table. Therefore, the spinal column is centered in an almost fixed location for *all* patients.

    The information that is stored in this level (with information type in parentheses) follows:

1. Distance between the centers of two organs (geometric attribute).

2. Whether or not two organs are touching each other (predicative attribute).

3. Whether or not one organ is included in the other (predicative attribute).

4. Type of tissue that lies between the two organs (quantitative attribute).

5. Tolerance in the distance between two organs (geometric attribute).

6. Whether or not there is an organ between two other organs (structural attribute).

3.5.3 Organ Level

Attributes associated with the organ level are:

1. A transformation to interface the organ geometry to the top level. This transformation is based on the location of the organ center relative to the body, and the orientation (rotations around the organ's origin). Therefore, this association is the $[x,y,z]$ coordinate of the organ's center in terms of the whole body and a 4×4 orientation matrix (geometric attribute).

2. Tolerance for the center point. Presents the uncertainty in locating an organ in the body (geometric attribute).

3. Organ size. The dimensions of an enclosing box for the organ. It consists of width, depth, and length in reference to the organ's coordinate system (geometric attribute).

4. Organ size tolerance. Presents the uncertainty in organ size (geometric attribute).

5. Typical CAT number for the organ (quantitative attribute. Restricted tool [see 1.4]).

6. Typical CAT number for the surrounding tissue (quantitative attribute. Restricted tool [see 1.4]).

7. Expert procedure that will control and manipulate the knowledge stored in the organ model, as well as collecting and processing solutions to goals presented to its descendants' model elements (the cross sections) (strategic attribute).

8. Modification expert routine that will carry out organ-level modifications (phase 3 of 3.4.2) (strategic attribute).

9. Description of lower level details of the organ shape and control, which is a link to lower levels of the model, i.e., the appropriate Generalized-Cylinder (structural attribute).

3.5.4 Cross-section Level

The cross-section level is associated with:

1. Center location of the cross section in respect to the organ's coordinate system (geometric attribute).

2. Tolerance for the center location (geometric attribute).

3. Cross-section size (geometric attribute).

4. Tolerance of cross-section size (geometric attribute).

5. Cross-section expert routine (strategic attribute).

6. Cross-section modification expert-routine that will carry out phase 3 (3.4.2) for this level (strategic attribute).

7. Cross-section descriptor, which is a uniform cubic B-spline planar curve to which the lower levels of the model are attached, defined in terms of the cross-section coordinate system. This is the link to the next, and last, model level (structural attribute).

The collection of center locations for all cross sections of an organ is the set of control knot points through which the main axis of the organ model is interpolated. The space orientation of the cross sections is defined by the shape of that main axis, which together with the cross-section center-point location defines the geometric transformation (T_c in Figure 3.2) to interface with its organ-level father element (see Appendix F for details). This geometric interface is recalculated at need (i.e., is not stored as part of the model). A descriptor of the cross-section shape is a uniform closed planar cubic B-spline curve. Such a curve is shown in Figure 3.2C. The curve is defined relative to the cross section's coordinate system. The curve definition is a list of control points along its periphery. Each of the control points is associated with the data concerning the fourth level (see next subsection). An additional potential geometric attribute is the cross-section rotation in its plane. This attribute is not listed here, since it is not used in this work.

3.5.5 Boundary-point Level

The information for the boundary-point level is:

1. Location of the boundary point in terms of the cross-section coordinate system (geometric attribute); and

2. Expert routine that will process and analyze the image in the vicinity of the cubic curve *segment* adjacent to its location (strategic attribute).

The collection of boundary points is the set of control knots for the definition of a B-spline curve (cf. Appendix B). Each boundary point controls an appropriate segment of that curve (shown saturated for P_1 in Figure 3.2C). When a boundary-point expert is activated, it will conduct searches at several points (the distance between which is determined at the cross-section level) along the adjacent curve segment. At each such point, the 2-D image of the cross section is searched for a boundary. The search is performed along a straight line, normal to the curve at this point and of a limited length that is also determined by the cross section. Each such search is considered an activation of an element of the boundary level and, being done along a straight line, the search is considered 1-D. The geometric interface between an element at this level and the cross-section level is calculated on need. The coordinate system for the boundary-point level is the path along which the image is searched. $\vec{CS}(t)$ is the planar vector-valued parametric curve that outlines the corresponding cross section. A boundary point is located at $\vec{CS}(t_0)$ for some t_0, so that the axis of its coordinate system is centered at that location, co-planar with the curve, and has a slope α,

$$\frac{\partial}{\partial t}\vec{CS}(t) = \left[\Delta_X, \ \Delta_Y\right] \tag{3.4}$$

$$\alpha = atan2(\Delta_X, \ \Delta_Y)$$

where $atan2(a,b) = tan^{-1}(a/b)$, in the appropriate quadrant.

The interface transformation (T_b in Figure 3.2) is defined to rotate around the origin of the cross-section coordinate system by α, and translates in X and Y by $\vec{CS}(t_0)$.

3.6 Chapter Summary

This chapter presented a hierarchical tree model that consists of four levels representing the knowledge, mainly geometric, about the domain in question, i.e., the human abdomen. The top level represents the gross anatomy of a collection of organs, each of which organs is a Generalized-Cylinder. The model is hierarchically decomposed through its levels in a method termed "shape refinement." All model elements in the various levels are shown to have some problem to solve (i.e., a goal), all of which problems are analogous to each other, though gradually decreasing in geometric complexity and dimensionality for the lower levels.

By understanding a 3-D image we mean finding the exact shapes of objects represented in it. This process is done by first creating a model-instance, then iteratively matching it with the data and modifying its shape until the fitting criteria are satisfied. The model tree structure is amenable to a highly parallel execution of this fitting scheme.

Two basic paradigms that underlie the fitting process are the *goal/subgoal paradigm* and the *modification paradigm*. Both are intuitive, both fit well with the hierarchical tree model structure, and both are powerful heuristics in matching complex 3-D shapes to 3-D data. *Expert routines* are specific procedural knowledge associations with model elements which are responsible for executing these heuristics, using the declarative knowledge stored in the model, especially the geometric interfaces between relating model elements.

4

Implementation and Applications

The SAIL programming language and a PDP10 computer have provided the implementation environment for this study. SAIL (Stanford Artificial Intelligence Language) is an ALGOL-like language that offers a rich variety of powerful data types, and an associative store called LEAP [Reiser, 1978]. LEAP has provided the building blocks for implementing the associative network for representing the whole model—especially that of the top level for gross anatomy. The language SAIL, its data types and specifically the LEAP associative store, as well as the possibilities for representing the relational knowledge for the gross anatomy as an associative network are presented in Appendix G.

The decomposition of a goal into its subgoals is the first basic computational paradigm (3.4.3); it is applied and implemented as the *search application and results propagation,* that is, phases 1 and 2 of the fitting process (3.4.2); and it implies a highly parallel process. The process of collecting results from lower levels, termed *result propagation* (phase 2 in 3.5), employs statistical tools for error-relaxation by out-liers detection and rejection.

The second paradigm is exercised by making hierarchical fitting decisions and is implemented as the *shape modifications.* The gross anatomy is consulted so that the organ-fitting criteria are satisfied first. Then small-scale changes are made in the cross-section level. Finally, when the cross-section level criteria are satisfied, the fit ends at the control points level.

Implementing the model as a network of associations is undoubtedly very flexible, enabling an intelligent program to replace, eliminate, and augment the model with new elements, depending on run-time conditions. Such new elements can be created at every level, can add more expressive power for shape details, or even generate "new" organs. For example, "new" organs that represent tumors will aid in locating them in the image.

This chapter discusses also the important issue of confidences at the result-propagation phase, search iteration convergence, and pyramid data organization.

4.1 Model Representation

4.1.1 Declarative Associations

The model is a set of items, each representing an organ. An organ item has a name (i.e., a PNAME) that corresponds to its biological name (e.g., "Spinal Column"). Each organ node is associated with organ-level attributes. Attributes for the top level are generally associated with more than one organ, e.g., pairs.

The associations for an organ can be defined in one of two ways: either at run-time by *making* them, and allocating all the needed data structures, or by restoring a LEAP dump from a file. At the same stage in which organ nodes are created and associated with their attributes, interorgan nodes, termed *NEIGHBORHOODs*, are established, with their appropriate interorgan attributes. These techniques allow the generation of the two top levels only. The other levels are composed of a set of hierarchical structures for the GC's of individual organs. These structures can be created in run time or "off-line" in a separate program. Our choice is to define them separately and save them in appropriate LEAP dump files.

When a model is stored in files, its overall structure is

$$< Model\ file> \atop < Organ\ file_1>,\ < Organ\ file_2>,...,\ < Organ\ file_N> \qquad (4.1)$$

The names of the appropriate files for individual organs are associated with the organ items. Organ "initiation" brings into memory the appropriate data structures and resolves all links. This particular choice of representation lets the definition of the "hairy" details of GC's be done separately.

Part of the system "initiation" is the generation of a *model instance*. To begin, the instance is an exact copy of the model geometric properties, which will be updated subsequently during the fitting process. At any stage during that fitting process, the whole model can be saved in files similar to Structure 4.1, by using a files-directory separate from that of the original model.

4.1.2 Expert Routines

Expert routines are treated differently from the declarative portions of the model. They are composed of an executable code that has to be compiled and loaded with the rest of the code in the program. When an expert routine is declared in the main code of the system, it is associated with a *generic* item that has a system-wide unique name (via a PNAME). The appropriate model node for which that procedure is the expert routine has also an association with the same generic item. When the model is created, or restored from files, these items are linked to resolve the dynamic association of an expert routine with a model node. In this way, the model can be edited in an environment that does not have the actual code for the expert routine, and the expert routine can be changed at will without the need to update the model accordingly. In the general case, the attachment of an expert routine to a model node is carried out via the following two triples:

$$\text{EXPERT-ROUTINE } of \text{ N } is < Generic_i >$$

$$\text{ROUTINE } of < Generic_i > is < Some\text{-}Item_j >,$$

(4.2)

where N is a model node, $< Generic_i >$ serves as the linkage "hook," EXPERT-ROUTINE is the attribute item for associating a model item with that "hook," and $< Some\ Item_j >$ is an item to which the appropriate routine is *assigned* and which is associated with the appropriate "hook" via the ROUTINE attribute. To apply an expert routine, one would use the following code:

$$apply(\text{Expert!Of(N), Parameters!Of(N)});$$

where Expert!Of(N) is a routine (or a compile time macro) that will first access the item $< Generic_i >$, as the first item in the derived set,

$$\text{EXPERT-ROUTINE } of \text{ N}$$

and then return the first item in the derived set,

$$\text{ROUTINE } of < Generic_i >.$$

The parameters for the application of the expert routine are retrieved in a similar way.

For purposes of efficiency, there is an exception to this arrangement in the boundary-point level. Elements of this level, which represent the control-knots of the spline definition for the cross-sectional curve, are stored in an array, where each row is a pair of coordinates. Corresponding to that array there is another array of items that contains expert-routine generics for the dynamic linkage of a node in the fourth level to the appropriate routine.

Figure 4.1 schematizes the model structure via all the involved types of sets, lists, and associations.

Figure 4.1   A schematic of all the data structures that participate
in the definition of a model, the various kinds of lists,
sets, and associations.

$\langle$ Model–Item $\rangle$ =

$$\left\{ \langle \text{Organ–Item}_1 \rangle, \langle \text{Organ–Item}_2 \rangle, \ldots \langle \text{Organ–Item}_N \rangle \right\}$$

for $i = 1, \ldots, N;$

$$\left[\langle \text{Organ–Attribute}_j \rangle \underline{\text{ of }} \langle \text{Organ–Item}_i \rangle \underline{\text{ is }} \langle \text{Organ–Attribute–Value}_{i,j} \rangle \right]$$

for $j = 1, \ldots, M; \quad i = 1, \ldots, N;$

$$\left[\text{ORGAN–SHAPE} \underline{\text{ of }} \langle \text{Organ–Item}_i \rangle \underline{\text{ is }} \langle \text{Organ–Shape–Item}_i \rangle \right]$$

for $i = 1, \ldots, N;$

$\langle$ Organ–Shape–Item$_i$ $\rangle$ =

$$\left\{ \langle \text{Cross–Section}_{i1} \rangle, \langle \text{Cross–Section}_{i2} \rangle, \ldots \langle \text{Cross–Section}_{iO} \rangle \right\}$$

$$\left[\langle \text{Cross–Section–Attribute}_l \rangle \underline{\text{ of }} \langle \text{Cross–Section}_{i_k} \rangle \underline{\text{ is }} \langle \text{Cross–Section–Attribute–Value}_{l,i_k} \rangle \right]$$

for $l = 1, \ldots, P; \quad i = 1, \ldots, N; \quad i_k = i_1, \ldots, i_O;$

$$\left[\text{SPLINE–VALUE} \underline{\text{ of }} \langle \text{Cross–Section}_{i_k} \rangle \underline{\text{ is }} \langle \text{Spline–Coefficients}_{i_k} \rangle \right]$$

$$\left[\text{EXPERT} \underline{\text{ of }} \langle \text{Generic–Expert}_h \rangle \underline{\text{ is }} \langle \text{Expert–Item}_h \rangle \right]$$

for $h = 1, \ldots, Q;$

$$\left[\langle \text{Organ}_{g_1} \rangle \underline{\text{ of }} \langle \text{Neighborhood}_g \rangle \underline{\text{ is }} \langle \text{Organ}_{g_2} \rangle \right]$$

for $g = 1, \ldots, R; \quad g_1, g_2 \in (1, \ldots, N);$

$$\left[\langle \text{Pair–Attribute}_f \rangle \underline{\text{ of }} \langle \text{Neighborhood}_g \rangle \underline{\text{ is }} \langle \text{Pair–Attribute–Value}_{f,g} \rangle \right]$$

for $f = 1, \ldots, S; \quad g = 1, \ldots, R;$

Where:

N	is the number of	Organs,
M	is the number of	Organ–Attributes,
i_O	is the number of	Cross–Section in the i-th organ,
P	is the number of	Cross–Section attributes,
Q	is the number of	Expert–Routines,
R	is the number of	Inter–Organ relations,
S	is the number of	Inter–Organ relation attributes;

Figure 4.1   (continued)

and

Tokens in   < ... >   **are item variables;**

Tokens in   < ... >   **with the key-word attribute or generic have unique PNAMEs.**

Upper-case tokens are unique PNAMEs of items.

$$\left\{ \langle \ldots_1 \rangle, \langle \ldots_2 \rangle, \ldots \langle \ldots_N \rangle \right\}$$ is a set or a list.

$$\left[< > \underline{of} < > \underline{is} < > \right]$$ is an association.

4.2 Search Application

4.2.1 General

The search application implements the goal/subgoal paradigm (4.4.3). Algorithm 4.1 schematizes the subdivision of a problem at some node into subproblems that are applied to descendant nodes, if there are any. Those nodes return a set of solutions which are manipulated collectively to provide a solution at the given node. The steps needed in this operation involve calculating the geometric interface to the next level, which is then concatenated with a transformation for the current level (passed to it by its "father"—its activator). The concatenated transformation is the key for aligning the activated node with its subimage (see 3.4.1) and enabling that node to work independently on achieving its own goal.

Algorithm 4.1

comment current!node is the node within whose environment this algorithm is executed. This node uses *current!trans* to transform its geometry to the body coordinate system, i.e., it is a 4 × 4 matrix of real numbers;

foreach node *such that* node *is* son *of* current!node
    do begin
            real array interface [1:4, 1:4];
            Find!Interface (node, interface);
            Concatenate (current!trans, interface);
            apply (Expert!Of(node),
                       { interface, image, ...});
      < collect results>
    end;
< apply modifications >;

where { ...} represents a list of *reference items*.

Parallelism. The total independence of descendants nodes permits their parallel application simultaneously. In SAIL terminology, the *apply* statement in Algorithm 4.1 is changed to

$$sprout(\text{node}, apply(\text{Expert!Of(node)}, \{ \text{ ... } \}));$$

In this way the item *node* becomes a representative of the *sprouted* process. The process of the activated node must then wait for the termination of all these processes by

$$join \; (\{ \; node_1, \; node_2, \; ..., \; node_N \});$$

where the set of nodes contains all those that have been *sprouted*. After all individual processes have terminated, the modification decisions can be made.

Depending on the level of the activating node, the various statements in Algorithm 4.1 are implemented differently. These statements are:

- Selecting of the next *node* in the *foreach* statement.

- Calculating the geometric *interface*.

- Retrieving the activated node *expert*.

The following subsections provide details of these implementations.

4.2.2 Top Level

For this level *node* is an organ item, all of which items are stored in a *set* so that the *foreach* statement is used directly:

$$foreach \; \text{organ} \; such \; that \; \text{organ} \; in \; \text{model} \; do \; ...$$

The geometric *interface* and the *expert* are associated with the given organ item, making possible their direct retrieval from the LEAP associative store.

4.2.3 Organ Level

In this level *node* is a cross-section item. Items here are stored in a *list* so that the *foreach* statement can retrieve them in order. The geometric interface is *calculated* by the method described in 2.3.3 and Appendix F.2 as the solution to the inter-cross-section orientation problem. The nature of this calculation is that it is done collectively for all cross sections of the GC of an organ, stored in a set, and retrieved from it in the body of Algorithm 4.1. The *expert* of a cross section is retrieved via a LEAP association.

4.2.4 Cross-section Level

A descendant node of this level corresponds to a point of the B-spline curve definition. Two parameters are provided by an expert of the cross-section level: one is *Step!Size*, and the second one is limit. 'Step!Size' corresponds to the density of application of fourth-level experts along the curve periphery.

The cross-sectional curve is made of *segments*, each enclosed by *control-knots*; each control-knot has a corresponding expert. The curve is considered to be a continuous curve divided equally by a set of *application points* into pieces, each of size *Step!Size*. If we have K such application points and O segments, then for each *application-point$_i$* there will be some *segment$_j$* in which it resides. The location of *application-point$_i$* and the normal to the curve at that point are used to calculate the *interface*. The *expert* of *application-point$_i$* is the one attached to the corresponding control-knot of *segment$_j$*. Under these circumstances, the *foreach* statement of Algorithm 4.1 turns into a *do* block over the number of application points. The generation of application points is accomplished through a special device called *stepper*, which is a data structure that represents all information about a *current* point on the cross-section curve on which it operates. Three operators are defined for a stepper:

- *Reset!Stepper* to reinitiate it,

- *Next!Step* to update it to the next point that is of some arbitrary distance (e.g., *Step!Size*) from the current one, and

- A predicate *End!Of!Stepper* to tell whether the whole curve has been completely traversed.

In addition there are the routines that generate a stepper *(Initiate!Stepper)* for a particular B-spline curve, and those that can retrieve from it the location *(Get!Location)* and normal *(Get!Normal)* vectors for the current point. The stepper may be introduced into Algorithm 4.1 by:

Algorithm 4.1.1

comment CS is a cross-section node.

```
stepper:= Initiate!Stepper ( CS);
Reset!Stepper (stepper);
while not End!Of!Stepper ( stepper) do
    begin
```

<activate expert for current application point>

...

Next!Step (stepper, Step!Size);
end;

Parallelism

In order to sprout a bunch of boundary point processes in parallel, new items must be allocated to be associated with activations of boundary point experts, which will be released after a corresponding *join* statement.

4.2.5 Boundary Level

At this level there are no subsequent nodes, with the result that Algorithm 4.1 for this level consists only of the <collect results> portion. An activated boundary expert routine at an application point searches in the vicinity of the CS curve. The search space per element is limited to a 1-D subspace of the 3-D image. Figure 4.2A is a plot of such a search: crossing the (cross-sectional) boundary curve is the line along which the image is searched. The graph in Figure 4.2B is of the image values along this line, where left-to-right corresponds to inside-to-outside motion along this line.

When moving along a straight line that crosses the organ boundary, one would expect the image values to change from those that correspond to the inside, to something different that corresponds to the outside. The expert in the boundary level has access to the information stored in the organ model and can retrieve that knowledge as the *Tissue!Of(organ)* and *Surrounding!Tissue!Of (organ)*. Potential boundaries are located where the density values change abruptly. A gradient transformation of an image is a very common way to find boundaries in 2-D images. In the 1-D analog presented here, the gradient is simply a derivative of the original 1-D function of image values vs. locations along the search line. Figure 4.2B shows an example of using the *gradient expert.*

Other experts are the *Pattern-Matcher* expert, which tries to match some 1-D pattern to the image function based on expectations, and the *Don't-Care* expert, which permits the discarding of some of the boundaries that are expected to be obscured and unreliable. The freedom of allocation of expert routines around a CS curve provides the indispensable capability to anticipate a variety of boundary conditions which a single procedure cannot handle.

4.2.6 Summary

The collection of all applications at the fourth level, per cross section, presents a dense coplanar search inside a narrow band along a planar curve. When

Figure 4.2   A) The positioning of the search line relative to the
               cross section and the image; and B) A gradient expert
               looks for the peaks in the differential (trivial gradient)
               of the 1-D image that present a function of the image
               values vs. location along the search line.

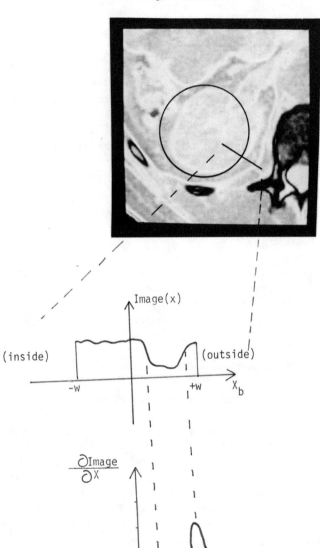

A.

B.

applied to all cross sections, the total application of fourth-level experts comprises a search inside a thin "skin" of a closed 3-D shape. This relation is demonstrated in Figures 4.3 and 4.4, for the cross-section level and the full 3-D image, respectively.

4.3 Propagation of Results

4.3.1 General

An important part of the results returned by any expert at any level is its *confidence* (a number between 0 and 1) in them. The confidence of the fourth- (1-D) level experts depends on how much the image (where they searched it) meets their expectations for the existence of an object boundary. On higher levels, this confidence is a function of the confidences returned by the descendants, and is discussed in detail in Section 4.3.6.

In the following subsections we survey the various ways for collecting and processing results at each level. We proceed from the lower levels upward, as shown in Figure 3.1 for the "results" arrows.

4.3.2 Boundary Level

On this level, the result is a 1-D coordinate in the reference system originated at the current boundary location, so that it reflects the *distance,* along the normal to a cross-section curve, of the newly found boundary from the current one. A positive distance is outside the corresponding cross-section; a negative distance is inside.

4.3.3 Statistical Tools

The ensuing sections make intensive use of statistical tools that are presented here.

The collection of results returned by the activated descendant nodes of the current one consists of some numerical geometric values which are tagged with confidences. They are considered a population of measurements for some random variable for which we wish to calculate the mean value. Some individuals of this population will be tagged with a very low confidence, and some (though they may have high confidence tags) will simply diverge widely from the main body of the population. We wish to calculate the mean value as the weighted average of the confident members (i.e., those which are tagged with high confidence, higher then some pre-set threshold) of the main body of the population. This process is known in the statistics literature as the rejection of out-liers [Natrella, 1963]. Here we use a procedure closely related to those proposed in the literature, termed here *Selective!Mean.* Figure 4.5 depicts the

Figure 4.3   The complete application of fourth-level experts by
              the cross section "covers" a narrow band around the
              cross-sectional curve, which is the model-instance for
              this level.

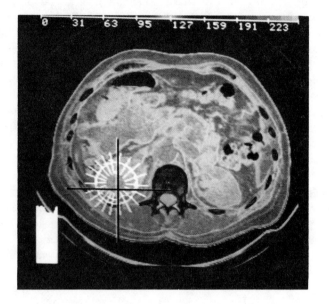

Figure 4.4   By applying the hierarchical search, the final result is
              one of searching inside the thin "skin" of the 3-D
              shape, defined by the geometry of the current model-
              instance.

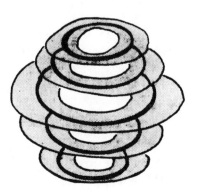

situation. It is a histogram of some measurements on a discrete domain, where the height of the function is the number of equally valued measurements. The letter μ is the algebraic mean of the total population which is not nonconfident, v^- and v^+ are some *factor* of σ away from μ, where σ is the standard deviation of the same population that was used to calculate μ; v^+ and v^- designate what portion of the population is rejected as out-liers, and μ' is the mean value of the remaining confident members of the population. That μ' is calculated as the weighted average based on the confidence tags of the given measurements. The value of *factor* in cases where the population is of size 10-20 is proposed in the literature to be about 3 (and it is so chosen here) when the measured random variable is of Gaussian distribution.

The algorithm for *Selective!Mean* takes as input five parameters: {A} is a set of measurements (the population), {Conf} is a corresponding set of confidences (i.e., $Conf_i$ is the confidence of A_i), Vf is the factor used to reject outliers, Gt is a threshold so that A_i is nonconfident if and only if $Conf_i < Gt$, and *Neutral* is the result returned if the population is not "clustered enough"(as will soon be explained). A *Neutral* value depends on the application; for a scale factor calculation, it is 1; for translation or displacement it is 0. Like Gt, there is also a threshold that determines whether a population is "clustered enough." It operates on the percentage of the population that is confident, i.e., not rejected as out-liers. *Selective!Mean*({A}, {Conf}, Vf, Gt, Neutral) is calculated in four steps as follows:

(SM1)   Let {A'} = Exclude({A}, {Conf}), to exclude from {A} all elements that have low confidence (designated by Gt).

(SM2)   Let M({A'}) and S({A'}) be the mean and standard deviation, respectively, of {A'};

(SM3)   Define {A"} to consist of all elements A_i' in {A'} that satisfy

$$|A_i' - M(\{A'\})| < Vf \cdot S(\{A'\}).$$

(SM4)   If [Size ({A"})/ Size({A})] $< Gt$, then {A} is not clustered enough, and Selective!Mean is set to *Neutral*. Otherwise, it is the weighted average of {A"}, where weights are corresponding selected confidences from {Conf}.

Note here that a "clustered enough" set {A} means satisfaction of the test in (SM4) for some values of Vf and Gt. Also, the last three parameters will be omitted in the subsequent text from "calls" made to Selective!Mean.

Figure 4.5   Calculating Selective!Mean. The letter μ represents the mean value of both the confident and out-lier regions; v^- and v^+ are some factor of σ away from μ, where σ is the standard deviation of μ and μ' is the newly calculated weighted average of the confident population only, where weights are confidences.

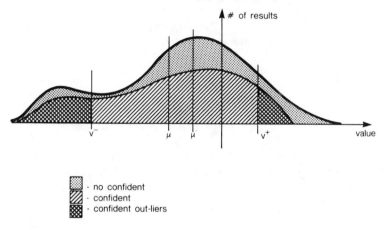

- no confident
- confident
- confident out-liers

4.3.4 Cross-section Level

An expert of the cross-section level collects 1-D results from all along the curve and converts them to 2-D with a geometric interface. Altogether there are two lists of 2-D coordinates, $\{[X_o, Y_o]\}$ and $\{[X_n, Y_n]\}$, and a list of numerical confidences, $\{Conf\}$—all in correspondence with each other. $[X_o, Y_o]_i$ is the old coordinate of the i-th application point, of which $[X_n, Y_n]_i$ is the new coordinate found by the corresponding expert, for which $Conf_i$ is the confidence. New values are computed as follows:

$$Dx_i = (X_n - X_o)_i$$
$$Dy_i = (Y_n - Y_o)_i$$
$$Distance_i = \sqrt{(Dx_i^2 + Dy_i^2)}$$

(4.3)

("Distance" is essentially the original result returned by the boundary expert.)

Changes to the cross-section shape are (affine) transformations that are considered in ascending order of difficulty: first, translation; second, scaling; and third, deformation (uneven scaling).

Translation. If $\{Dx\}$ and $\{Dy\}$ are clustered enough, then the curve location is translated by Selective!Mean($\{Dx\}$, $\{Conf\}$) in the X direction and by

Selective!Mean({Dy}, {Conf}) in the Y direction, only if the amount of translation is greater than a given fraction of the voxel size of the searched data.

Scaling. If {Distance} is clustered enough and Selective!Mean({Distance}, {Conf}) is greater than a given fraction of the data resolution, then the curve is scaled around its center by the factor

$$\frac{Selective!\,Mean\,(\{\,Distance\}\,,\{\,Conf\})}{< Curve-Diameter>},$$

where <Curve-Diameter> is defined as

$$Maximal\ [(Max(\{X_o\}) - Min(\{X_o\})),$$
$$(Max(\{Y_o\}) - Min(\{Y_o\}))].$$

Note that no transformations or changes are made, but only suggestions are propagated to the organ level together with confidences in them.

4.3.5 Organ Level

The expert in the organ level considers data of a 3-D nature that is limited to the close vicinity of the volume occupied by the organ. The decisions made at this level are much more complicated than those at lower levels simply because of the higher dimensionality involved.

A cross-section element returns

1. [Dx,Dy] and Disp!Conf, the displacement suggestion for the cross section and its confidence in that result, respectively, and

2. [Sx,Sy] and Scale!Conf, the scale suggestion for the cross section and its confidence in that result, respectively.

These geometric results are transformed to the appropriate organ coordinate system via a geometric interface. After applying the transformation we get four lists: {[Dx,Dy,Dz]} with the corresponding {Disp!Conf}, and {[Sx,Sy]} with the corresponding {Scale!Conf}.

Figure 4.6 presents several examples of the type of processing possible with these results to come out with changes at the organ level, i.e., in 3-D.

Translation in X-Y-Z. We first calculate the following values:

$Org!Dx = Selective!Mean(\ Dx\ ,\ Disp!Conf\ ,...)$

$Org!Dy = Selective!Mean(\ Dy\ ,\ Disp!Conf\ ,...)$ $\qquad\qquad$ (4.4)

$Org!Dz = Selective!Mean(\ Dz\ ,\ Disp!Conf\ ,...)$

Figure 4.6 Five cases in considering changes in the organ level geometry for the model-instance based on the collection of results from the cross-section levels. A-B) Displacement in the X-Y-Z directions and scale in the X-Y directions, respectively, based on all-agreed suggestions by the cross sections. C-D-E) Based on the divided opinion of cross sections at both ends, the organ is translated (C), or scaled (D,E) in Z.

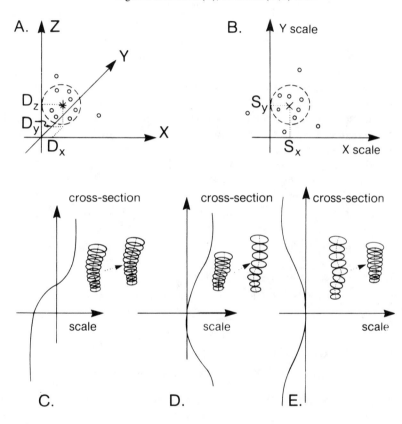

If the sets {Dx}, {Dy}, and {Dz} are clustered enough with respect to the corresponding confidence sets, and |[Org!Dx, Org!Dy, Org!Dz]| (i.e., the size of the 3-D displacement) is greater than some fraction of the voxel size of the image (finer than which is useless to try to get), then this change is suggested and passed to the top level, as shown in Figure 4.6A. This change means that first we would like the organ model to be positioned in the center of the searched organ before the other, more complicated, changes are tried.

Scale in X-Y. In some cases, the cross sections are approximately parallel, so that scaling in their X-Y direction corresponds well to scaling in the X-Y direction of the whole organ. When the searched organ displays such characteristics (e.g., the kidneys), then the following calculations and change suggestions are tried (Figure 4.6B):

let
Org!Sx:= Selective!Mean ({Sx}, {Scale!Conf},...)

Org!Sy:= Selective!Mean ({Sy}, {Scale!Conf},...)
(4.5)

If the total change in the organ size by these scales does not exceed some fraction of the data resolution, then it is excluded.

Translate and scale in Z. Any change in the Z direction is more complicated to reach than such changes in the X-Y directions. To suggest a change in the Z direction, the collection of 2-D results from the cross sections is divided into two groups, one at each end of the organ object, that are analyzed separately.

Limited to 2-D, the individual cross sections cannot perform or suggest modification that involves 3-D reasoning, which is therefore based on the aggregation of results from a set of such 2-D entities.

We divide a given list of results, {G}, into two groups, {Top!G} and {Bot!G}, each consisting of results from a corresponding portion of the cross sections. In our case, {G} stands for either of {Sx}, {Sy}, {Dz}, {Disp!Conf}, or {Scale!Conf}. Accordingly, we calculate representative values:

Org!Top!Sx:=Selective!Mean ({Top!Sx},{Top!Scale!Conf},...)

Org!Bot!Sx:=Selective!Mean ({Bot!Sx},{Bot!Scale!Conf},...)

Org!Top!Sy:=Selective!Mean ({Top!Sy},{Top!Scale!Conf},...)

Org!Bot!Sy:=Selective!Mean ({Bot!Sy},{Bot!Scale!Conf},...)
(4.6)

Org!Top!Dz:=Selective!Mean ({Top!Dz},{Top!Disp!Conf},...)

Org!Bot!Dz:=Selective!Mean ({Bot!Dz},{Bot!Disp!Conf},...)

Figures 4.6C and 4.6D represent the three possibilities:

1. Both Org!Top!Sx and Org!Top!Sy are positive, while both Org!Bot!Sx and Org!Bot!Sy are negative (or vice versa). This case arises when the cross sections at one end are too small, while those at the other end are too large (Figure 4.6C). In an organ that is egg-shaped, such as the kidney, this fact suggests translation in the Z direction depending on which end it is desired to expand. Such a change mimics the movement of an air blob in a jar of honey or that of a drop of water in a can of oil, and depends on the direction of the translation.

2. Org!Top!Sx, Org!Top!Sy, Org!Bot!Sx, and Org!Bot!Sy are positive (Figure 4.6D). In this case, it turns that the cross sections at both ends desire to expand. When an organ is known to have an egg shape, its expert is programmed to conclude from this that the organ-instance is too short, and suggests scaling in the Z direction (that approximates its longitudinal axis). The amount of scaling is not clearly derived from these four values, but in a step-wise approach; we scale by no more than about 5% to 10% in each iteration, to ensure convergence.

3. Org!Top!Dz and Org!Bot!Dz are opposite in signs. This suggests scaling in the Z direction, as shown in Figure 4.6E. These changes mean that the organ-instance is "pulled" or "squeezed" at both ends. The amount of scaling is, as in the previous case, by trying a step-wise convergence and scaling each time by a small amount.

The obvious advantage of the first basic computational paradigm (3.4.3) is demonstrated in particular when one considers changes at the 3-D organ level, as shown in this section. No individual cross section could suggest anything in the Z direction, since each is a limited 2-D entity, but the collection of cross sections is combined into a 3-D object, and, collectively, they can serve as a basis for conclusions in the 3-D aspect.

NOTE: This section constitutes basically an example of what can be done at the organ level. Its power rests in utilizing the *collection* of 2-D results for a 3-D conclusion. Different domains will require different approaches, but within the framework set forth here.

Vertical scanning. As can be observed from Figure 4.4, the searches conducted by the cross sections are biased toward the planarity of cross sections and do not provide a good indication of how the organ fits the data in the vertical direction. The organ-level modifications that try to infer a translation or scale in Z have to use data that is closely oriented parallel to the X-Y plane. In cases where the organ has also distinguished top and bottom (such as a kidneys), it is desirable to conduct a search at the organ level that will look in a direction lined up by the main axis at both its ends. This is vertical scanning, since it is perpendicular to the scans made by the two end cross sections. Such scans, it becomes evident, are major contributers to change suggestions in the organ's Z direction (Z is considered the vertical direction for the organ).

4.3.6 Confidences

Until now we have not said much about the way the confidences are calculated. It is very important that one not be too confident, but it is also important not to be over-suspicious. At each level, an appropriate method is applied to calculate confidences.

At the boundary level the appropriate method depends on how much the image displays the expected characteristics of an organ boundary, given all the knowledge concerning the typical organ tissue CAT numbers and the surrounding tissues CAT number, and taking into account the fact that the search at this level is conducted from *inside* the organ to its *outside* (assuming that it begins close enough). (See also next subsection.) At this level, confidences are very specialized to the particular expert. The *gradient-expert,* for instance, will measure the abruptness of change in image values, triggering the sensation of an organ boundary. The strongest confidence occurs when the image values change from those typical of the organ interior to those typical of its surroundings; the weakest confidence occurs when the image values are too far from those expected. Another use of confidences is demonstrated with the *Don't-Care* expert that always returns confidence 0.

At the cross-section level we are presented with a collection of results of searches along the periphery. The basic tool to deal with these results is the *Selective!Mean* that operates under some parameters and thresholds. Intuitively, if most results are not confident enough, this cross section cannot come to any confident conclusion. If they are all very confident but contradictory (reflected as not being "clustered enough"), the same effect occurs: the cross section still has weak confidence at any conclusion that it will come upon. In general, the *Selective!Mean* algorithm provides a very good measure of confidence, which is the test in (SM4) for the fraction of "good" results in the total collection. Therefore, at the cross-section level, confidence depends on the number of "good" boundary searches out of the total conducted along its periphery.

At the organ-level a similar rationale as for the cross-section level is used to infer organ-level confidence based on results from cross sections and their associated confidences.

4.3.7 Errors Relaxation

In all three levels of result propagation, the retrieved results are never totally reliable and can cause errors if this unreliability is not taken into account.

Results propagation begins with the simple and, seemingly, trivial boundary experts. They search raw data which are strange (noisy and obscured) enough to allow them to consider mistakenly the wrong result as a very confident one. Most of the results will not be so misleading or, when not accurate, will be accompanied with a low confidence. For this latter reason, some of the boundary experts will be the *Don't-Care* expert that will always return results with no confidence, to be ignored later, in places were data is expected to be unreliable. Also for this reason, experts operate on very well-defined and restricted subimages out of the whole image.

An indispensable condition for the successful convergence of the fitting process is that only a relatively small portion of the experts' applications is radically erroneous. Being so, the statistical filtering of *Selective!Mean* ignores the more divergent (out-liers) results, basing conclusions on a cluster of "good" results. This assumption is justified if the initial conditions for the search are satisfied, i.e., that the initial instance is a close approximation to the actual anatomy. As already mentioned, for some of the organs we can be very confident as to their location in the image (e.g., the spinal column that is naturally always centered in the back). That fact emphasizes the importance of knowledge about gross anatomy that relates to the image those less distinguishable organs (e.g., kidneys) via the "easier" organs.

Another important assumption is that the vertical (longitudinal) positioning of the patient is sufficiently accurate. Although that positioning in the scanning machine is done manually, it can be assured by strict regulations to be carried out by the scanner technicians.

4.4 Modifications

All that the search experts did at each level was to provide *suggestions* for changing the model-instance to improve its fit with the data. Suggestions at each level are recorded by attaching them to the appropriate model element, since they may be attended some time later (during the third phase).

After results have been propagated to the top level, the modification phase starts. It begins with modifying organs as 3-D objects. Later, cross sections of individual organs are modified, and so forth. Modifications are accomplished by experts that are attached to model elements in exactly the same way as the search experts. There are modification experts at each level that (when activated) retrieve the appropriate stored results from the model and examine them for compatibility with the model geometry constraints. The improved results are then used to modify a model element.

As long as there are required changes at a given model level, no further changes are made to lower levels (thus conforming to the second basic paradigm given in 3.4.4. As long as the organ can be changed as a 3-D rigid body, as a 3-D shape, etc., by translating and scaling it, no additional modification will take place. When no more changes at this level are required (when the search experts find nothing to do), the fitting criteria at that level are considered to be satisfied. At this point, the modifying experts of the descending model elements are activated.

Once the fitting criterion at a given level is reached, the fit may be lost again by subsequent modifications at lower levels, thus requiring modifications to recur at higher levels. As a whole, this modifications scheme corresponds to the three-phase fitting process as described in Chapter 2.

4.5 Pyramid of Resolutions

The 3-D image consists of a large amount of data, far too large for the machine capacity of the PDP10. However, most of the organs occupy small subimages. In the pyramid-of-resolution approach (cf. processing and image cones in [Hanson, 1976; Tanimoto, 1978]), the system starts with a coarse resolution of a large portion of the data (actually all of it). Being at a low resolution (i.e., every voxel represents a large volume in the domain), there are few enough voxels to pose no memory constraints. When the model is matched against low-resolution data, some organs may be too small to be satisfactorily located. In any case, organ shape and location cannot be updated to a better accuracy than some fraction of the voxel size (for example, 0.5).

When all search opportunities in the image at a given resolution are exhausted, the organ location is much more restricted and constrained, so that the next round of matching is done in a subimage containing the organ, in the next level of finer resolution, as depicted in Figure 4.7. The details of implementation and representation of multiresolution images are provided in Appendix D.3.

Figure 4.7   Application of the pyramid-of-resolution principle: after the organ is located in the coarse resolution that consists of a large portion of the image (volumetrically), the surrounding volume (smaller) is accessed in a finer resolution (more voxels per unit of volume), and then the same practice is repeated until the finest resolution image possible (resolution factor 1) is searched (see Appendix D.3 for the definition of resolution factors).

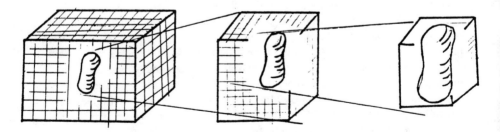

Section 1.6 discusses the benefits of *scanning planning* as a utilization of the scanner in stages, making use of its ability to scan in several possible resolutions. The data in this study were provided in the highest possible resolution and have been artifically converted to lower resolution data by an averaging technique. In an actual environment, the low-resolution data will be acquired directly from the scanner and are expected to be free of the additional artifacts of the averaging process used here. The averaging effect can be visualized in Figures D.3 and D.5.

4.6 Modification Convergence and Constraints

When one analyzes the fitting process, one cannot avoid asking the questions: "How stable is the process?" and, "How can one assure convergence?" If we follow the principle of ordering shape modifications according to their complexity, what if the organ starts "swinging" between two locations unstably, trying to converge (for example) the translation modification, and never succeeds, though a scale modification could help it? These problems are aggravated by the fact that the data are discrete, and the "grains" (voxels) of which the image of a smooth organ is made are large enough to be problematic when fine shape modifications are needed. To answer these problems, a more elaborate scheme is presented and its implementation is given, while an even more general approach is discussed in 6.4. The solution chosen here is to add *stabilizers* to the convergence process and to use more shape constraints for modifications.

A very simple stabilizer for converging a numerical process is to pose a limit on the number of iterations allowed. A more elaborate stabilizer is one that looks at the history of the process and decides when it starts "dangling" between two semistable states. This stabilization is accomplished by associating each node with an archival storage of all changes suggested in the last *generation* of, say, five iterations. If the average change in the last generation is less than a given threshold, then the last change is ignored. The result is an apparently stable process that converges (though with the help of an external mechanism).

The Generalized-Cylinder concept itself imposes some shape constraints on the organ geometry and will constrain modifications of individual cross sections. When a cross section is translated by changing the 3-D coordinates of its center, it redefines that main axis shape and, as a result, the shape of the whole organ. It is desired to keep the organ model physically feasible and prevent cases like that shown in Figure 2.8A. For this reason, the main axis shape defines constraints on the allowed translation of cross sections, consequently limiting that type of modification in this level. The underlying formula is developed in Appendix F.3; the method assures a "discrete

Generalized-Cylinder" through curvature constraints. Independently of that, the organ size and organ center location and tolerances limit the possible modifications in the organ level and cause the modification process at this level to converge. The fitting process consists of three types of iterations:

1. *Organ Iteration:* the iterations that are executed until the organ level criterion is satisfied. When satisfaction occurs, the cross sections are activated and modified as individual 2-D problems, constrained by the global organ shape.

2. *Cross-Section Iteration:* the iterations that allow each cross section to solve its individual 2-D problem.

3. *Major Iteration:* a complete cycle of an organ-iteration and all the subsequent cross-section iterations.

This process is controlled by limiting the number of these iterations and using stabilizers. It operates as described in the following algorithm:

Algorithm 4.2:

for MI:= 1 *step* 1 *until* Major!Iterations
    do begin "major iteration"
        logical Major!OK, Organ!Modified, CS!OK, CS!Modified;
        Major!OK:= *false;*
        Organ!Modified:= *false;*
        for OI:= 1 *step* 1 *untl* Organ!Iterations
            do begin "organ iteration"
                <activate organ>
                if <satisfied> *then*
                    begin "organ satisfied"
                        Major!OK:= *not* Organ!Modified;
                        done "organ iteration"
                    end "organ satisfied";
                <modify organ>;
                Organ!Modified:= *true*
            end "organ iteration";

        CS!OK:= *true;*
        foreach cross!Section
            do begin "cross section"
                CS!Modified:= *false;*
                for CSI:= 1 *step* 1 *until* CS!Iterations
                    do begin "cross section iteration"
                        <activate cross!section>;
                        if <satisfied> *then*
                          begin "cs satisfied"

```
            CS!OK:= not CS!Modified and
                  CS!OK;
            done "cross section iteraton"
          end "CS satisfied";
        < modify cross section>;
        CS!Modify:= true
      end "cross section iteration"
    end "cross section";
  Major!OK:= Major!OK and CS!OK;
  if Major!OK then
      done "major iteration";
end "major iteration";
```

In this algorithm, the statements for activating, satisfaction, and modification of the various model elements mean as follows:

<satisfied> is true when the suggested changes by the corresponding element are too small for the given image resolution, or that the stabilizer operating on that element have eliminated any farther changes.

<apply> is the activation of a node expert.

<modify> is the activation of a node modifier.

To summarize, the fitting process invokes in each iteration all the model hierarchies from a given level and below, until all elements of that level are satisfied, and then goes to search and modify the next lower level. When modifying a given element, mechanisms such as stabilizers and numerical limitations help bring the process under control.

5

Examples

5.1 General

Three levels of examples are provided that correspond to the lower three fitting levels (cf. Figure 3.1). The first example is a set of pictures (Figure 5.1) of the 1-D searches at the boundary level, along the boundary of a cross section. The other two examples are for the analysis of a 2-D image and a 3-D image. The second example presents a smaller scale fitting problem than for the 3-D problem, but provides a sizable demonstration of the fitting strategy. The fitting problem is solved iteratively. For the 2-D case, the model consists only of two levels that correspond to the *cross-section* and *boundary-point* levels (cf. Figure 3.1). The search, results propagation, and modifications as explained in the previous chapter are iterated over these two levels only.

In the 3-D example, a 3-D object is searched. Here the model consists of three levels, including the *organ* level. This third example concentrates mainly on operations at the organ level.

5.2 One-Dimensional Example

Each of the pictures in Figure 5.1 demonstrates a search normal to the boundary of a cross section. The function of image values vs. distance from the model boundary is plotted on the bottom left of the screen. After all searches along the boundary are completed, the effect is of searching a narrow band along the model boundary.

5.3 Two-Dimensional Example

In fitting the circular model for the cross section of the left kidney, the search starts somewhat away from the center of the organ. A series of pictures is shown in Figure 5.2 for some of the iterations taken until the process converges. Each picture displays the current model imposed over the analyzed image and the fixed coordinate system relative to which the model is changed. The coordinate system represents the initial model position. On the right, the three

Figure 5.1   One-dimensional search example.

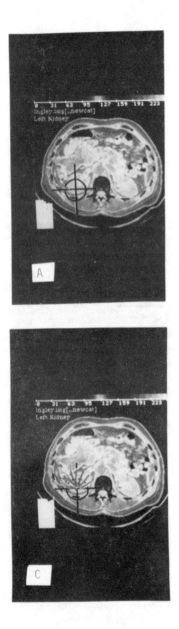

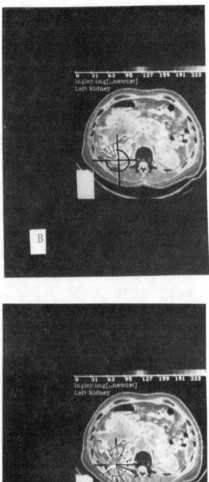

histograms represent (from top to bottom) Distance, Displacement along the X direction, and Displacement along the Y direction (see discussion in 4.3). The banner on the bottom announces the modification decision.

The role of error relaxation (cf. 4.3.7) is the most important characteristic of the fitting strategy that can be learned from this example: as the model converges to the correct location, the aggregated results from the boundary experts cluster more and more, showing greater agreement with fewer misleading results. In spite of the errors and large divergence during the first iterations, the aggregated result is still the correct one.

5.4 Three-Dimensional Example

In this example (Figure 5.3), the left kidney is the object of the search, and the 3-D model instance is modified according to the discussion in 4.4. The series of pictures concentrates on iteration at the organ level. There are two groups of pictures, the first one (plates A-D) constitutes the stages in fitting the left kidney of one patient, while the second group (plates E-J) presents the final results of other organs and of other patients as well. The pictures stand as follows:

A. A shaded graphics view of the models for the two kidneys and a portion of the spinal column.

B. The initial location of cross sections of the model relative to the image. The cross-section curves are plotted over a 2-D image of the corresponding cross section of the 3-D image. The order of the plates corresponds to the Z order of cross sections from top to bottom.

C. Changes in the organ level during the fitting process. In these pictures, a vertical cross section of the 3-D image at the center location of the organ model serves as the background. On this 2-D image, the 3-D organ model is projected, including a projection of the main axis (blue curve) and the cross-secion curves (white curves). The 3-D orientation of the organ is depicted by the projection of the X and Z axes of its own coordinate system (yellow and orange). The changes are evident when observing these plates in order from left to right, top row, and then bottom row.

D. The final situation at the end of the fitting process as reflected in the position of cross-section curves, relative to the image. This series of plates is similar to A above, and shows how well the final model-instance fits the actual organ.

Figure 5.2   Two-dimensional fitting example. A) Initially, the
              model instance is far from the correct solution and
              the returned results are largely scattered, with many
              erros. B) After a few iterations, the model approaches
              the correct solution, and the results cluster more,
              while the errors decrease.

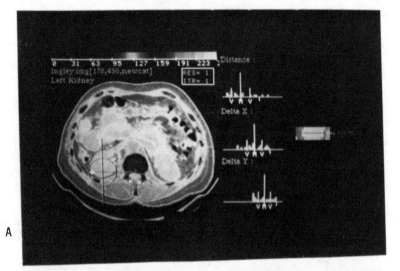

A

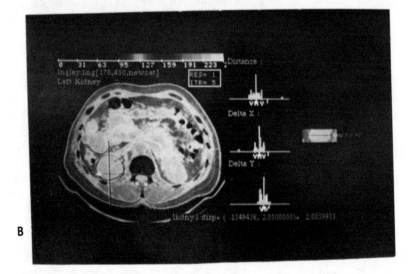

B

C) Results clustering increases. D) Finally, the results cluster in the middle and the model fit exactly on the object (amid local changes along the boundary).

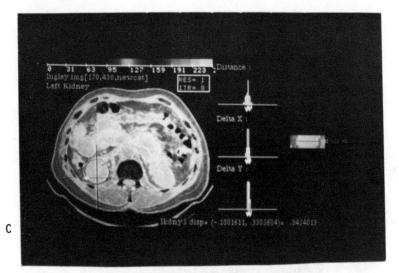

C

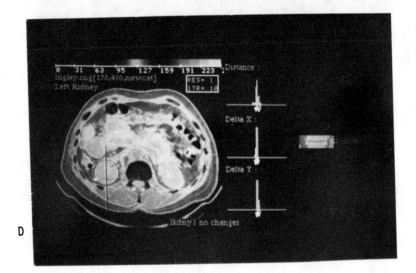

D

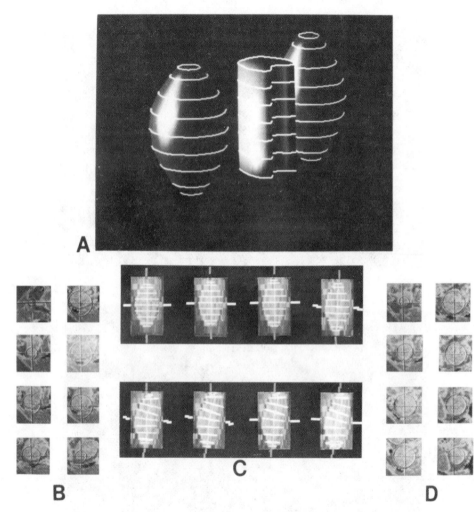

Figure 5.3   Three-dimensional fitting example.

Figure 5.3   (continued) Three-dimensional fitting example.

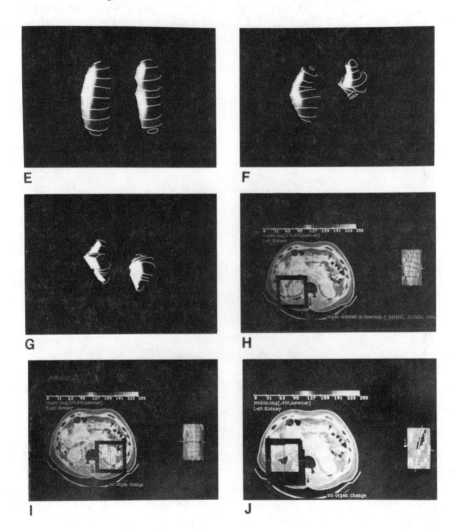

E-F-G.   A shaded graphics display of the final model-instance for both the left and right kidneys, for the first, second, and third data sets, respectively.

H-I-J.   A view of the final situation in fitting the left kidney of the first data set, the right kidney of the same data set, and the left kidney of the second data set, respectively. Each image shows the display layout during the system run when the the graphics option is ON. The left portion of each image is the X-Y view of the organ coordinate system, with the 2-D cross section of the image, and the plot of a cross-section curve from the model-instance. On the right is the X-Z projection of the model-instance as it was for plate B above.

To complete this example, one should refer to the trace listing of the fitting process in Appendix E.

6

Summary and Conclusions

6.1 General

The ideas presented in this study have not evolved in a vacuum but have been heavily influenced by a school that believes in model-driven, rather then bulky data-driven, approaches to vision problems. Experiments in knowledge-based image analysis in the Computer Science Department of the University of Rochester have proved the validity of the approach and its advantages. Ballard [Ballard et al., 1978; Ballard, 1982] has built a system for the detection of ribs in chest radiographs, in which the knowledge was imbedded in a network of experts and strategists that evaluated the cost of applying image operators (edge detectors, boundary followers, and so on) and their applicability at each point. This idea was further developed and formalized as "constraint networks" [Russell, 1979]. Constraint networks provide the tools to define a model for an image; the model is then applied to "constrain" the image regions where a feature might be located. The network is built of strategists and experts, each tagged with its cost and effectiveness, and each of which may be invoked depending on the state of the analysis. This technique was used for outlining docked ships and sewer tanks in aerial photographs, as well as for detecting ribs in chest radiographs.

Because analyzing 3-D images with 2-D techniques may not work, a model-directed and knowledge-based approach seems more promising even though it imposes hard and new problems (see also the introduction and Chapter 1). A first attempt in this direction was made by Schudy [1980] for detecting the heart in ultrasonic scans: a highly parameterized model of spherical harmonics surface is fitted to the shape of the actual heart in the image. Not many other projects of this kind are known; the closest one is that of Soroka [1979; 1981], who used generalized-cones as primitive geometric-shape models that were combined into higher order 3-D shapes, guided by a centralized production system for inference-making. No other known projects used any high-order knowledge but, rather, approached the problem bottom-up (i.e., they were "data-driven"). [Liu, 1977; Rhodes, 1979]. Both Liu and

Rhodes applied well-known, semiautomatic 2-D image analysis techniques, namely boundary-following and region-growing, respectively, and extended them to 3-D (in Liu's case, even 4-D).

The technique presented in this thesis captures the problem in a very general way. It assumes that the data is a 3-D structure with no bias to the scanning orientation of a particular CAT-scanner, and it uses powerful geometric-shape modeling based on Generalized-Cylinders. Knowledge is decentralized, and appears everywhere in the model as procedural experts and data. The problem of fitting a shape model to the data is hierarchically controlled and concentrates on solving local problems by the experts. This technique is extendible to other applications where *a priori* knowledge is at hand, by using tools (made available here) to build a model and specializing experts for best performance.

6.2 Achievements and Future Work

This section reassesses the most important of the accomplishments listed in the introduction. The preceding chapters discussed the various aspects, techniques, data structures, principles, and paradigms involved in this research, and demonstrated an actual test of them on three data sets.

As shown in the examples of the previous chapter, the system performed with about 50% success. We argue here that the lack of consistent knowledge and the change in scan conditions of the given data sets are at the root of the problems encountered.

6.2.1 The Fitting Process

The backbone of this work is the fitting process; its success is bound to the decomposition of a complicated 3-D fitting task to simpler components of lower dimension in a hierarchical way. Hierarchies are integral to this approach— in the iterative fitting process and the data structure of the model and its experts. The principles of combining the various components of model and problem for a solution are provided by two intuitive and simple computational paradigms. Notable about the fitting process are the following facts:

1. *Real data.* The system is tested on actual CAT scans of random patients of the Strong Memorial Hospital, Rochester, N.Y. (the only criteria for choosing them was their being abdominal scans of 10 mm interslice distance and their lack of contrast agents. The last condition could not be fulfilled for all data. Real data is in contrast to CAT scans of phantoms or the computer simulation of scanned phantoms [Simmons, 1978].

2. *Convergence* of the fitting process. The forces involved in modifying a model shape to fit some other data shape are widely diverse and will not stably converge unless special mechanisms are applied.

3. *Speed* of convergence is high when the full parallelism option is utilized, making the time for a full iteration on one level equivalent to the iteration time in a single element of the next level below, plus some small overhead.

4. *Solution to a hard problem: "find the kidneys".* Finding kidneys is undoubtedly difficult in comparison to locating other organs that are more distinguishable from their surroundings. Solving this problem was stated earlier as one of the reasons for preferring this model-driven approach over data-driven ones, of which several systems already exist.

The results of the three tests in the previous chapter have demonstrated good performance for both the left and right kidneys of the first data set. The left kidney in this first data set was used during the debugging phases of the system, but not the right kidney. The other data sets differ from the first one in several aspects: the corresponding patients took contrast agents prior to the scan, the scans were slightly less dense (i.e., larger interslice distance), and the second data set showed "stones" in the kidneys. The system located the kidneys correctly, although it showed confusion about their correct shapes. The analysis of the fitting process for these tests revealed a large proportion of erroneous and uncertain results at the boundary-level experts. These results were too poor to make a sound, correct decision in the higher levels, though still good enough to pass the confidence-threshold tests, thus preventing the system from *admitting* failure.

6.2.2 Generalized-Cylinders

The development and exploitation of the Generalized-Cylinder had not been fully accomplished prior to its application to this project. This powerful tool, as demonstrated here, could not have been available without the adoption of spline techniques from computer graphics and CAD. When compared to other, more restricted, uses of GC's, the use made of this tool in this project is a large step forward.

6.2.3 Scene Interpretation

In solving any vision problem, a most important question is whether or not the scene is interpreted by the analyzing program. It is generally the task of a separate stage of the program that tries to compare results to some catalog of shapes (cf. [Marr & Nishihara, 1976]). In this thesis, the interpretation is "free" and implicit, since objects are located by name and not by the arbitrary location of some initial point in space. When one wants to find the left kidney, he types: "Find left kidney." In any event the program always produces interpreted results.

6.2.4 Loose ends

The main efforts were concentrated in the organ and cross-section levels and omitted some of the important problems in the gross anatomy at the top level and in modifications at the lowest level, the boundary level. In the intermediary levels, only a restricted set of shape modifications was developed and applied. These present problems will form the base for future research.

Intermediary levels. In the cross-section level only displacement and scaling were tried. Problems arose when a nonflexible circle-shaped model was fitted to an ellipsoidal object in the image. More general theories and techniques are due here, as well as a more rigorous mathematical discussion of the definition of "best fit," and the proof that it is available. The same applies to the 3-D level, or organ level, although the additional dimensionality makes the introduction of theories and mathematical rigorousness more complicated and more demanding, but very challenging.

Boundary level. In respect to searching the data in the boundary level, the boundary experts were far simpler than one could make them, and they were allowed to make errors far too often. These experts analyzed a 1-D subimage as a 1-D image, though they could access it as a 1-D subimage of a 3-D image, utilizing a powerful 3-D gradient [Zucker, 1979]. On the other hand, modifications at this level were avoided altogether, though they could provide an exact fit and full details of the object's surface. There is still work to be done as to the way in which individual results of the boundary experts can change the shape of a cross section locally—for instance, by increasing the number of spline control points.

Top level. The top level is intended to provide a good starting position for the process of fitting a particular organ, based on relational knowledge. The gross anatomy will also restrict the changes in shape of an organ and prevent it from "wandering" too far and getting lost, and will use locations of already discovered reliable organs (e.g., the spinal column) to locate the softer and more obscured organs like the kidneys. Relational knowledge is very useful when it is reliable and available, which, unfortunately, is not always the case. There is a need for a significant and larger scale penetration of computers into the world of medicine and health care. One of the prospective contributions of this work is the introduction of the importance of computerized medical data-bases for anatomical interference-making for relational knowledge which is useful in analyzing CAT images. However, medical application is just one field where this technique is applicable. In industry, mechanical parts inspection is a promising field, since the descriptions of such parts are well cataloged and all geometrical knowledge is available, possibly in digitized form.

The top level can be useful in yet another way—by generating "new" organs, for the purpose of discovering anatomical defects and tumors: one of the uses of CAT scans in medicine is to discover such cases, frequently by noting changes in the expected locations of visible organs. The same reasoning that lets the diagnostician deduce the possibility of a tumor can be based on results provided by this system and the use of gross anatomy, anatomical data-bases, and a sophisticated inference-making mechanism. When the location of a tumor is thus predicted, it can be further searched by generating a model for an artificial object, the tumor, and starting a search for it. The process of locating a tumor can be aided by reactivating the CAT-scanner for a better resolution in the locations indicated.

6.3 Comparisons

6.3.1 Taxonomy

The prominent projects in the field of 3-D image analysis will be compared, based on the following criteria:

1. *Results representation:* Whether results representation is parameter-ized or bulky. A parameterized result is more convenient for further processing and shape analysis, besides being compact. Whether the results are interpreted.

2. *Strategy:* Whether the image is analyzed bottom-up or top-down and whether it is data-driven or a model-driven, respectively.

3. *Control:* Whether the image is analyzed via a centralized control or the analysis control is decentralized to allow local control of the search for individual features.

4. *Weaknesses:* What the main problems with the approach are, and how well the method performs on various types of data.

5. *Operation mode:* How much the analysis can be automated and freed from the intervention of a human operator.

6.3.2 Comparisons with the Literature

The most important works in the analysis of 3-D images are also largely in the medical area and have been reported by [Soroka, 1979; Liu, 1977; Rhodes, 1979; and Schudy, 1980]. These projects are aimed at providing a geometric representation of objects in 3-D images. Soroka, Liu, and Rhodes deal with CAT scan data, while Schudy uses ultrasonic scans of the heart. These projects are compared in Table 6.1 with the work presented here with regard to the categories above.

Table 6.1.   A Comparison of the Important Research Projects in Understanding 3-D Images with the Work Presented Here.

Researcher	Representation	Structure and Control	Operational Characteristics
1. *Soroka*	Parameterized combination of generalized-cones. Uninterpreted.	Centralized control via a production system. Bottom-up approach. Image is analyzed on availability.	Vulnerable to noise and artifacts in data. Automatic, ries to find everything in the image. Image is conceived as a collection of stacked parallel slices.
2. *Liu*	Objects are a collection of boundary voxels. Not parameterized, but bulky. Uninterpreted.	Data-driven, bottom-up approach. Searching for boundary by a 3-D boundary-following technique. Algorithmic approach.	Vulnerable to noise and artifacts in data. Good only to distinguish objects like the lungs and bones in medical CAT scans. Semi-automatic, user must point at starting point. Image is a 3-D data structure
3. *Rhodes*	Collection of voxels in interior of organ. Not parameterized, but bulky. Uninterpreted.	Data-driven, bottom-up approach. 3-D region-growing technique. Algorithmic approach.	Vulnerable to noise and artifacts in data. Good only to distinguish objects (like bones or lungs). Semi-automatic, user must point out a "seed" voxel in the image. Image is a collection of stacked parallel slices.
4. *Schudy*	Parameterized shape as a spherical harmonic surface. Interpreted.	Top-down, model-driven, centralized conrol. Data is searched on need only.	Image is a 3-D data structure. Automatic fitting of model to object. Objects must be functions on a sphere.
5. *Shani*	Parameterized by generalized-cylinders. Interpreted.	Top-down, model-driven, decentralized control. Image is searched on need only. Makes use of pyramid-of-resolution image organization.	Image is a 3-D data structure. Automatic fitting of a model to organ of choice. Organs must have a longitudinal axis, or be decomposed to a collection of such objects.

6.4 Fitting as a Case of Searching

In artificial intelligence (AI) terms, the fitting process is viewed as searching in a multidimensional space. In this view, there are two important notions: that of *states* and that of *state evaluation* [Winston, 1977] when the goal is to reach a state whose value is minimal (or maximal). The dimension of the search space is determined by the number of independent parameters needed to define a state; in our case it is the number of different types of modifications that are allowed. If modifications are continuous (as is the case here), then the number of states is countless. In the examples in Chapter V, and from previous chapters, only two kinds of modifications are considered here: *scale* and *translation*. The evaluation function measures how much a given model instance fits with the feature to be located in the image, shown in the shaded areas in Figure 3.3. A continuous-search space is easily converted to a discrete space by allowing only fixed (small) modifications at a time, of each type.

Given this interpretation of the problem, any of the many search strategies in common use in AI can be employed. If the evaluation function is expensive, we would do better to use heuristics in choosing the set of next-best potential states to be evaluated, and so forth. Backtracking is a necessity in searches, when a chosen path leads to the wrong way.

The approach taken in this study is an extreme case where heuristics and evaluation functions play a major role in eliminating and minimizing the number of considered states in every step. In fact, only one state is examined at a time, and only one type of modification is applied at a time. The evaluation function is expressed in the results returned by an expert and serves as the basis for a calculated guess (heuristic) as to the best modification to be applied. A compromise between the adopted strategy here and the AI view would be to try to *look ahead* and examine several possible next states, evaluate them, and choose the best. This process may result in a combination of modifications (i.e., simultaneous scale and translation), replacing the heuristic approach, as described in the second basic computational paradigm (cf. III.4.4).

In any of these possible approaches, AI categorizes such a search as "hill climbing," and calls for a more careful consideration of the local search space before taking the next step in the direction of the hill-top—the solution that will maximize the fit (or minimize the difference, as provided by the evaluation function). Experience with the system shows that when one modifies the instance, large steps should be avoided, since this "hill climbing" approach means that a path to the solution may have been missed. In all the given examples, only small modifications were applied at a time, even if the heuristics could justify a large step.

6.5 Conclusions

The work is far from done. Two significant points have been left out: one is the extensive use of relational knowledge and the other is the accurate fit of boundary points to the data. Relational knowledge is very useful when it is available and reliable—both of which are, unfortunately, not true yet in the medical application field. However, the application of this technique to mechanical parts inspection, for instance, is very promising since top-level knowledge is quite handy.

Although relational knowledge is important, it is not a crucial condition, as the results in the given examples have shown. A more important problem is to further exploit the possibilities in shape control and changes of the model, or even find other means to model 3-D shapes. In the case of Generalized-Cylinders, we did not try to deform cross sections or even to scale them unevenly, and we did not allow detailed changes in the lowest level of the boundary point, that could make the instance exactly fit with the actual data.

Appendix A

CAT Scans

A.1 Introduction

In 1895, Wilhelm Konrad Roentgen excited the world with the discovery of X-rays. Soon radiology became an integral part of diagnostic medicine, a necessary tool in any medical institution of any size. It provided diagnosticians with a view of the inside organs of the body by projecting them on a plane as if they were objects of various transparencies.

In 1968, a new invention was registered in the London Patent Office by Godfrey Newbold Hounsfield [Hounsfield, 1972], in the name of the EMI Corporation; that was the first CAT-scanner (Computed Axial Tomographic Scanner), or as titled in the patent application:

"A METHOD OF AND APPARATUS FOR EXAMINATION
OF A BODY BY RADIATION SUCH AS X
OR GAMMA RADIATION."

The new technique was to scan an object plane-wise and to collect a large number of measurements of systematic and accurately planned radiation rays through it, and with the aid of a computer, to reconstruct the internal structure of the scanned material. The result is a set of 2-D digitized images, one for each scan, the values of which are the *linear attenuation coefficients* for radiation absorbency of the corresponding material in the object, which is proportional to their *density*.

The first images that were thus obtained revealed the delicate structure of soft brain tissues, a view that is impossible with regular radiology. Since then, CAT-scanners have become necessary to any modern hospital. Several generations of scanners have evolved during the last decade in efforts to provide better quality images, faster scanning time, lower radiation doses, the ability to scan larger objects, and reconstructed images with higher resolution. The first operative scanner was a head-scanner that provided images of low 80 $\times$ 80 resolution, while the latest General Electric Company CT/T 8800 scanner is a body-scanner that provides images of resolution 320 $\times$ 320, of which each *voxel* can represent as small a volume element as $1 \times 1 \times 5$ millimeters. Figure A.1 is a picture of a scan taken by the CT/T 8800 scanner of the chest region. CAT scanning consists of three phases:

1. Collection phase, in which a large set of measurements is made and digitized;

2. Reconstruction phase, in which the huge amount of collected data is processed, to compute a reconstructed 2-D image; and

3. Image analysis, in which diagnosticians analyze the images, with some help from computers.

Figure A.1.   An example of a CAT scan of the abdomen made by the General Electric Company CT/T 8800 scanner.

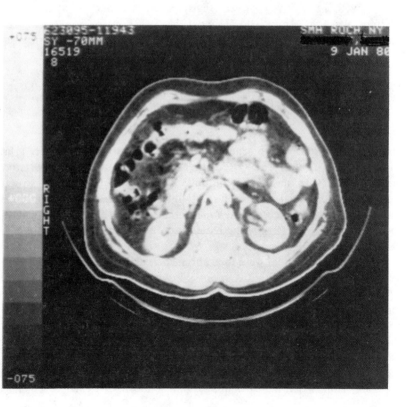

Every CAT-scanner provides the first two phases. The mathematical basis for the second phase has been of great interest to mathematicians since the turn of the century, but it could not be put to practical use before the introduction of computers. The main contributor to the mathematics of reconstruction, as employed in the CAT-scanner, is Allan M. Cormak, who shares with Hounsfield the 1979 Nobel Prize for Medicine for their contributions to the invention of CAT-scanners.

In this appendix, we present the operational principles for the first phase, and the mathematical background and reconstruction algorithms for the second phase. We also discuss some of the difficulties and problems with CAT reconstruction.

A.2 Operational Principles

The basic apparatus is shown in Figure A.2. It consists of a radiation source and a detector, one at each side of the scanned object. The object is scanned in the plane α (with a coordinate system X-Y). When centering a coordinate system on this plane, the source-detector line is denoted as $L_{k,\Theta}$. When a thin ray of radiation is emitted from the source, its initial level is I_o. The radiation is partially absorbed and scattered by the encountered material, and transmitted radiation of level I_d is detected. The relation between these two radiation levels lets us compute the *line-integral* $P_{k,\Theta}$ along the radiation path. When μ_t is the linear attenuation coefficient function of the scanned material, limited to the radiation path,

$$
\begin{aligned}
I_d &= I_o \exp\left[-\int (\mu_t \, dt)\right] \\
P_{k,\Theta} &= Log\left(\frac{I_d}{I_o}\right) = -\int (\mu_t \, dt)
\end{aligned}
\tag{A.1}
$$

$P_{k,\Theta}$ is also considered a projection along this line, and when this value is measured for a range of k, the whole plane is projected on a line, in a way similar to regular radiology for a whole volume, only here the values are discrete and digitized (cf. Figure 1.2)

When this process is repeated for Θ, varying from $0°$ to $180°$, the whole disk is covered by projecting the plane in all directions, as depicted in Figure A.3.

A similar effect can be obtained by *fan-beam* radiation of a single source that may be collected by an array of detectors, a process that is repeated in all $360°$ of directions. While the technique in Figure A.2 is typical to the first-generation CAT-scanners, later generations began to use a growing number of aligned detectors, working in parallel. More recently (and much more expensively) CAT-scanners utilize a large set of both sources and detectors for

Figure A.2. The line-integral $P_{k,\Theta}$ along the line $L_{k,\Theta}$ is measured, based on the source radiation level I_o and the detected radiation level I_d, and Eq. A.1

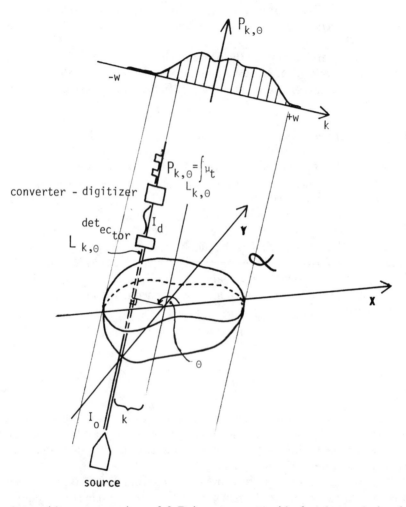

the rapid reconstruction of 3-D images to provide for the analysis of the temporal behavior of internal organs (e.g., the heart) [Riteman, 1979].

The collected measurements are passed to the second phase for reconstruction. There, the system of integral equations is solved for a discrete approximation for μ_t which is a matrix of values, $\mu_{i,j}$. Figure A.4 schematizes what happens. The scanned object portion is a slice of some thickness that is then divided into a matrix of *voxels*. Each voxel has some average attenuation

Figure A.3. When measuring $P_{k,\Theta}$ for $k = -w$ until $+w$, and Θ from 0° to 180°, the whole plane is projected in all possible directions.

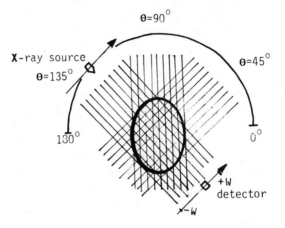

Figure A.4. Discrete integration for $P_{k,\Theta}$ is the summation over the attenuation coefficients $\mu_{i,j}$ of all the voxels that intersect the line $L_{k,\Theta}$, weighted by $A_{k,\Theta,i,j}$.

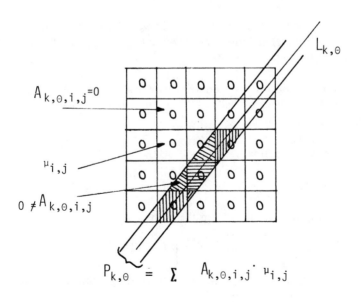

coefficient $\mu_{i,j}$. When radiation ray, $L_{k\Theta}$, penetrates through the object, it intersects some of the voxels in varying amounts, described by the matrix $[A_{k,\Theta}]$, where $A_{k,\Theta,i,j}$ is the portion of the i,j-th voxel that intersects with the $L_{k,\Theta}$ ray. The matrix $[A]$ is, obviously, very sparse. Together with the measured value $P_{k,\Theta}$, we get the equation

$$P_{k,\Theta} = \sum_{i,j} (A_{k,\Theta,i,k} \cdot \mu_{i,j})$$

(A.2)

As many such equations are obtained as there are measurements, i.e., for all k and for all Θ, yielding a huge system of linear equations to be solved. The system may be singular, or ill conditioned; it is simply too big to be sure about, so that a straight-forward Gauss elimination technique may prove insufficient. Therefore, it is solved differently, as will be described in the next subsection. What the above discussion provides is an intuitive hunch that the whole problem is solvable since there is enough data from the projections to reconstruct the internal, projected structure.

A.3 Reconstruction Methods

The reconstruction problem can be stated as follows:

Problem A.1:

For a function $f(x,y)$ on a plane, we are given all its line integrals $P_{k,\Theta}$. Can we evaluate $f(x,y)$ at some arbitrary point $p = [x,y]$ based on these line-integrals? If so, how?

If $P_{k,\Theta}$ is given for continuous k and Θ, then the answer is YES, as proven by the (already classic) work of Radon [1917]. The function $f(x,y)$ must obey the following conditions:

1. Everywhere defined;

2. Continuous;

3. Has a bounded integral on the plane

$$\int\int \left[\frac{f(x,y)}{\sqrt{x^2+y^2}} \right] dx \; dy; \text{ and}$$

4. For every point $p = [x,y]$, the circular integral of radius r around it converges to 0 for large r:

$$\lim_{r\to\infty} \left\{ \frac{1}{2\pi} \cdot \int [f(x+r\cdot\cos(\Phi), \; y+r\cdot\sin(\Phi)] \; d\Phi \right\} = 0$$

Let's define $F_p(q)$ as the circular integral of all line integrals $P_{k,\Theta}$, that are tangent to a circle of radius q around point p.

Now we can evaluate $f(x,y) = f(p)$:

$$f(p) = -\frac{1}{\pi} \cdot \int_0^\infty \frac{\partial F_p(q)}{\partial q}$$

$$= \frac{1}{\pi} \cdot \lim_{e \to \infty} \left\{ \frac{F_p(e)}{e} - \int_e^\infty \left[\frac{F_p(q)}{q^2} \, dq \right] \right\} \tag{A.3}$$

In practice, we are confronted with a discrete and finite version of the problem: $P_{k,\Theta}$ is given for only finite number of k-s and Θ-s. A solution for the practical, discrete, and finite problem was proposed by another classic work in this field [Bracewell, 1956]. It was for the reconstruction of the distribution of radio wave sources, based on aerial beam scans in radio-astronomy, which are strip integrals, i.e., the discrete version of line integrals that have some width.

A somewhat artistic reconstruction problem is discussed by Birkhoff [1956] to reconstruct a picture by drawing straight black lines of fixed width, and in all directions across a white paper. With respect to the terminology given at the beginning of this section, each straight line represents a line integral, $P_{k,\Theta}$, and the drawing is a *back-projection* of the line integral by dividing its value equally to all image points along it. While the drawn lines have fixed width, their density varies, which has the effect of lines with varying widths, or grayness (Figure A.5). This method became known later as the *Summation Method*, for which Birkhoff analyzed the nondigital (analog) solution; another analog solution [Kuhl & Edwards, 1963] has reconstructed a 2-D image by summing up back-projections on a cathode ray tube. Reconstruction techniques are divided into four main methods:

- The summation method;

- ART (Algebraic Reconstruction Technique);

- Fourier methods; and

- Convolution methods.

There are almost as many applications of reconstruction algorithms as there are serious researchers in the field, so that we shall try to present here a short, semiformal, description of the various algorithms. A good reference for this purpose is [Gordon et al., 1970].

Figure A.5. Birkhoff's drawing on a white paper with straight lines, that
is equivalent to simple back-projected discrete line integrals
(taken from "On Drawings Composed of Uniform Straight
Lines," by George D. Birkhoff, Journal De Mathematique,
Volume 19(3), 1940, page 235).

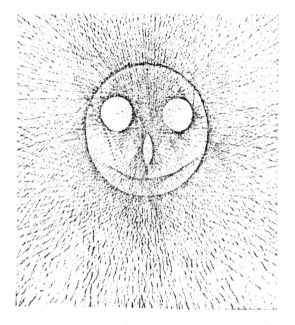

A.3.1 The Summation or Back-projection Method

We can invert the line-integrals given in Eq. A.2 by adding to each $\mu_{i,j}$ a portion
of $P_{k,\Theta}$, for all k and all Θ.

$$\mu_{i,j} = \sum_{k,\Theta} \left[\frac{P_{k,\Theta} \cdot A_{k,\Theta,i,j}}{\sum_{i,j}(A_{k,\Theta,i,j})} \right] \tag{A.4}$$

This technique is equivalent (within a scale factor) to blurring the image,
or convolving it with a certain point-spread function. In the continuous case
of infinitely many projections, this function is simply $h(r) = 1/r$, that is,
radially symmetric.

A.3.2 Algebraic Reconstruction Technique [ART]

This technique is an iterative solution to the linear system of Eq. A.2. The initial value of the image is

$$\mu_{i,j,0} = O; \text{ for all } i,j \tag{A.5}$$

At each iteration step, we calculate the line integral $P'_{k,\Theta,m}$ of the current image at the *m*-th iteration, and back-project the *difference* between it and the measured data

$$\mu_{i,j,m+1} = \mu_{i,j,m} + \sum_{k,\Theta} \frac{(P_{k,\Theta} - P'_{k,\Theta,m}) \cdot A_{k,\Theta,i,j}}{\sum\limits_{i,j} A_{k,\Theta,i,j}} \tag{A.6}$$

This method was employed in the first EMI CAT-scanner, providing very satisfactory results. The main drawback is its computational cost, which makes it infeasible for large images (such as the 320×320 images on the CT/T 8800 scanner). There are several versions of ART algorithms, of which the two most useful are the MART (Multiplication ART) [Gordon et al., 1970], which uses multiplication instead of addition in Eq. A.6, and the SIRT (for Simultaneous Iterative Reconstruction Technique) [Gilbert, 1972b].

A.3.3 Fourier Methods

Definition A.1: A central section of a function $f(x,y)$ is defined as $[S_\Theta f](R)$ to be the restriction of $f(x,y)$ to the straight line that passes through the origin with slope Θ

$$[S_\Theta f](R) = f\left(R \cdot \cos(\Theta), \ R \cdot \sin(\Theta)\right). \tag{A.7}$$

A basic theorem in Fourier analysis is

Theorem A.1: The Fourier transform of a one-dimensional projection of a two-dimensional function is identical with the corresponding *central section* of the two-dimensional Fourier transform of the original function.

Notationally, if we define $[P_\Theta f](R)$ as the continuous case of line integration in a given direction, Θ

$$P_{k,\Theta} = [P_\Theta f](k), \tag{A.8}$$

and $[F_n f]$ as the *n*-th Fourier transform of the *n*-dimensional function f, then Theorem A.1 states that

$$[F_1 P_\Theta f](R) = [S_\Theta F_2 f](R)$$
$$= [F_2 f]\Big[R \cdot \cos(\Theta),\ R \cdot \sin(\Theta)\Big] \qquad (A.9)$$

Now, the function $f(x,y)$ can be reconstructed by simple inverse Fourier transform:

$$f(x,y) = [F_2^{-1}\ F_2 f](x,y), \qquad (A.10)$$

where $[F_2 f](w,u)$ is found from either Eq. A.9, or by interpolating through values obtained by that equation.*

Therefore, the technique includes three steps:

1. Calculate $[S_\Theta F_2 f]$ for all $\Theta = 0°, \ldots, 180°$ based on Eq. A.9, from the measured $P_{k,\Theta}$, $k = -w, \ldots, + w$.

2. Based on these values, interpolate for $[F_2 f](w,u)$ for any arbitrary w, u.

3. Use Eq. A.10 to reconstruct $f(x,y)$.

Because of the data discreteness, only the discrete Fourier transform versions of Eq. A.11 are used. This method is quicker than the ART, since it is a "one-pass" technique, thus speeding up reconstruction of large images, and a Fourier transform can be done by FFT (Fast Fourier Transform). The main drawbacks are the vulnerability to errors through the repeated transformations and the interpolation phase, which is in addition to commonly expected errors in the data collection phase that precedes the reconstruction itself.

————————

NOTE

The Fourier transformation and its inverse are defined (for the 1-D case) as

$$[F_1 f](x) = \int_{-\infty}^{+\infty} \exp(-2\pi\, jxu)\, f(u)\, du$$
$$[F_1^{-1} f](u) = \frac{1}{2\pi}\int_{-\infty}^{+\infty} \exp(2\pi\, jux)\, f(x)\, dx \qquad (A.11)$$

where

$$j = \sqrt{-1}.$$

This technique can be applied with transforms other than the Fourier transform, too [DeRosier, 1971; Crowther & Klug, 1971].

A.3.4 The Convolution Method

This is the most popular method in current CAT-scanners, which combine Fourier techniques and the summation method. It is a *one-pass* technique, and by overcoming the blurring problem in the summation technique, yields excellent results.

The convolution method is the natural extension of the summation method. Recognizing that the summation method produces an image degraded by a convolution with some function *h,* it attempts to remove the degradation by a "deconvolution." The straight-forward way to accomplish this is to Fourier-transform the degraded image, multiply the result with some band-limiting function (to remove the high spatial frequencies), and inverse-Fourier-transform the result. Since all the operations are linear, however, a faster approach is to convolve the projections with an appropriate function to form a filtered set of projections, before performing back-projections. This method is faster since the convolution of the projection data is done during the data collection phase. To put it formally, we define the band-limited Fourier-transformed function $F'(w,u)$

$$F'(w,u) = [Ff](w,u) \cdot B(w,u) , \tag{A.12}$$

where $B(w,u)$ is 1 in a limited area around the origin, and 0 everywhere else.

The filtered reconstructed function is, therefore,

$$f(x,y) = [F_2^{-1}F'](x,y)$$
$$= \frac{1}{4\pi^2} \int_{-\infty}^{+\infty} \int_{-\infty}^{+\infty} F'(x,y) \cdot \exp(2j(wx + uy)) \; dw \; du. \tag{A.13}$$

By converting $[w,u]$ to polar coordinates $[R,\Phi]$, we get

$$= \frac{1}{4\pi^2} \int_0^{\pi} \int_{-\infty}^{+\infty} F'(R,\Phi) \cdot \exp\left(2jR \left(x \cdot \cos\Phi + y \cdot \sin\Phi\right)\right) \cdot | R | \; dR \; d\Phi. \tag{A.14}$$

We can convert $[x,y]$ to polar coordinates $[k,\Theta]$ too,

$$f(x,y) = f(x \cdot \cos\Theta + y \cdot \sin\Theta, \; \Theta)$$
$$= f(k,\Theta), \tag{A.15}$$

which means that,

$$x \cdot \cos\Phi + y \cdot \sin\Phi = k \cdot \cos(\Theta - \Phi).$$

By substituting the above conversions in Eq. A.14, we get

$$f(k,\Theta) = \frac{1}{4\pi^2} \int_0^\pi \int_{-\infty}^{+\infty} F'(R,\Phi) \tag{A.16}$$

$$\cdot \exp\left[2jRk \cdot \cos(\Theta - \Phi)\right] \cdot |R| \, dR \, d\Phi,$$

$$= \int_0^\pi g'\left[k \cdot \cos(\Theta - \Phi), \Phi\right] d\Phi,$$

where,

$$g'(L,\Phi) = \int_{-\infty}^{+\infty} [F'(R, \Phi \cdot \exp(2jRL) \cdot |R|] \, dR. \tag{A.17}$$

Clearly, Eq. A.16 is the back-projection of $g'(L,\Phi)$. If we define

$$H(R,\Phi) = |R| \cdot B(R,\Phi), \tag{A.18}$$

then Eq. A.17 is a convolution of $g(L,\Phi)$ and $q_\Phi(L)$, where $g(L,\Phi) = P_{L,\Phi}$ [*i.e.*, the projections of the original function $f(x,y)$ in direction Φ), and $q_\Phi(L)$ is the function shown in Figure A.6A.

As it turns out, filtering the Fourier transform of the function is equivalent to back-projecting the convolved projections by the function shown in Figure A.6B, which is the intuitive way to remove the blurring effect of simple back-projection and summation (see also the excellent discussion in [Brooks, 1975]).

A.4 Some Problems with CAT Scans

The CAT scan image is one of the best things that a diagnostician could ever have wished for; the images obtained by the machine are much superior to those first images more than ten years ago. However, CAT scans have some drawbacks; the major one could be their cost (close to a million dollars in 1980 prices). Some of the more technical problems are the time length that a single scan takes, the radiation doses induced in the patient, and artifacts in the reconstructed images.

Lengthy Operation

The time that a single scan takes may be long (minutes), and usually a patient is scanned 10-20 times. While taking a single scan, the data collected is assumed to have no time component. If a scan takes too long, movements of internal organs will cause errors in the reconstruction process. Recent generations of

Figure A.6. Convolution filters. A) The function $q_\Phi(L)$; and B) The convolution filter for back-projections.

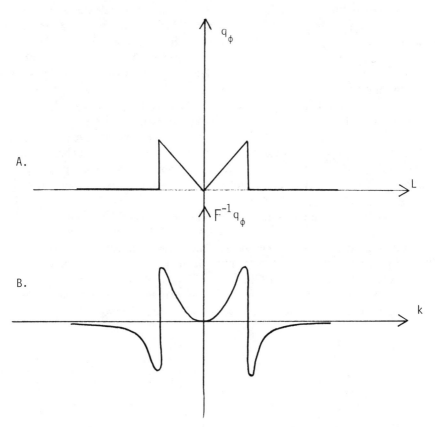

A.

B.

CAT-scanners have reduced greatly the elapsed time for the actual data collection phase for a single scan and put it on the seconds scale. Still, a single patient occupies the machine on the average for about 30 minutes. More modern machines (not commercial yet) will be fast enough to retain temporal information as well as 3-D images [Riteman, 1979].

Radiation Doses

CAT scans are not recommended for casual radiographic examinations because of the large doses induced in the patient. The number of slices (scans) influence this amount too. Recent developments, however, have reduced these radiation doses reasonably and eliminated most of the radiation hazard [McCullough, 1978]. Today, CAT scans are done even to newborns.

Artifacts

Reconstructed images may be degraded by artifacts, which are false features that appear in the image in addition to noise. Artifacts are due to mathematical ambiguity in solving the reconstruction problem, in the transition from the unique, continuous solution, to the approximated discrete one. Some of the reasons for artifacts are the sharp spatial changes in tissue density that cause discontinuities in the reconstructed function due to "aliasing." Sharp tissue changes exist at boundaries between bones and muscles, bones and fat, and at air pockets; their effect on the image is that of "cast shadows."

The scanning technology itself is the cause of another type of artifacts called *beam hardening* [Tsai, 1976]. The radiation is not monochromatic, of which the longer (and weaker) waves are absorbed and scattered more rapidly than the "harder" waves. This situation violates some of the basic assumptions of Eq. A.1.

Machine alignment is also a problem; each of the measurements of Eq. A.1 assumes that I_o is the same all the time, and that I_d is measured under the same conditions as for all other measurements. An array of detectors (as in the later generation CAT-scanners) must be repeatedly checked for detectors equivalence [McCullough, 1976].

A thorough survey of these CAT scan artifacts and others, like motion, partial volume, and so forth, can be found in [Goodenough, 1975].

Appendix B

B-Splines

B.1 Introduction

Spline theory has been explored in depth by numerous researchers and is summarized in many articles and books. It was first introduced by Schoenberg [Curry & Schoenberg, 1947], when it began attracting mathematicians and engineers. The main developments have been made during the last 15 years.

In the more general case, *finite element* methods have vastly contributed to this field; after the invention of the computer, nonanalytic solutions to differential equations became feasible. A solution space for a tough problem could be projected onto a comfortable space of piece-wise polynomials (PP) of a finite dimension. PP-s became an important tool in solving many engineering problems [Ciarlet, 1975].

A simple case of such a problem is to interpolate a univariate function through a large set of points (termed *knot points*) with the objective of finding an interpolant that is bound to some continuity and smoothness conditions. The classic interpolation with a single high-degree polynomial does not work very well: when the interpolation points are numerous, it suffers from computational inefficiency and instability. Following a finite-element approach, the interpolation problem can be "broken" into a collection of simpler interpolations of short segments. Altogether these segments will adhere to the interpolation conditions by providing the desired continuity and smoothness, also across "mesh" points where neighboring segments meet. Each segment is of a low-dimensional space, much lower than that required to solve the problem with a single analytic function. When each segment is interpolated by a polynomial, the interpolant is a PP. For the linear vector space of PP-s, B-splines are convenient basis functions, mainly due to their computational efficiency and their property of locality, which is a key feature in solving finite-element problems. The dimension of a PP space is the number of degrees of freedom in defining it, which corresponds to the total number of coefficients of its polynomial pieces. It depends on the number of knot points, the maximum degree of the polynomials, and the continuity conditions across knot points.

PP-s are very attractive for interpolating smooth curves in two (or three) dimensions, mainly in Computer Graphics and CAD/CAM (Computer-Aided Design/Manufacturing). It can be extended to surface interpolation as a tensor-product of such curves, a method known as "Coons Patches" [Coons, 1967; Forrest, 1972].

When dealing with curves, we represent them parametrically:

$$\vec{C}(t) = [X(t), \ Y(t)], \ t \ \epsilon \ (t_0, \ t_1), \tag{B.1}$$

when t is the curve parameter that may correspond to arc length. Both of $X(t)$ and $Y(t)$ are univariate functions of t, and are correspondingly, but individually, interpolated through the set of knot points $\{X_i\}$ and $\{Y_i\}$, so that the final curve will pass through the set of points $\{[X_i, Y_i]\}$.

The mathematical background for the theory of piece-wise polynomials with B-splines will be discussed in the next section. The rigorous mathematics can be found in a recent book [DeBoor, 1979]. The practical reader can refer to an important one of the many papers DeBoor has in this field [DeBoor, 1972].

In computer graphics *uniform cubic B-splines* are mainly used. Here each polynomial piece of a PP is cubic, and the curve parameter changes uniformly from piece to piece (or segment to segment), though not corresponding to arc length. They were first introduced into shape design and CAD/CAM by [Riesenfeld, 1973]. In Riesenfeld's work, the useful and well-known method of *Bezier curves* [Forrest, 1972] was shown to be a special case of *Variation Diminishing Uniform B-Splines,* which is an application of B-splines to approximation. This application will be discussed in a later section.

B.2 Piece-Wise Polynomials

Definition B.1: Piece-wise polynomial (PP)

Given a knot sequence $T = \{t_0, t_1, \ldots, t_n\}$, and a sequence of n polynomials of order k, $P_i(t)$, we define a piece-wise polynomial $P(t)$:

$$P(t) = P_i(t) \text{ for } t_{i-1} \leqslant t < t_i \tag{B.2}$$

$$(i=1, \ldots, n)$$

such that each of its pieces is a polynomial of order k.

We say that the polynomial $P(t)$ is in the space $P_{k,T}$ i.e., the space of all PP-s of order k over the knot sequence T. Figure B.1 is an example of such a polynomial. Note that there are no restrictions as to continuity across knot points.

Figure B.1.   A piece-wise polynomial.

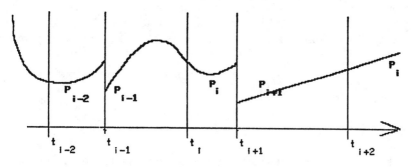

Any function $F(t)$ can be approximated by a PP $F'(t)$ as a linear combination of *basis functions*. For a given set of basis functions, the approximation $F'(t)$ is represented as a vector of coefficients, $\vec{V}$. The number of required coefficients, $|\vec{V}|$, is the dimension of the corresponding space of PP-s. The dimensionality is equivalent to the *number of degrees* of freedom in defining $F'(t)$. For the space $P_{k,T}$

$$Dim(P_{k,T}) = n \cdot k \tag{B.3}$$

for the reason that, for each of the n polynomials, there are k degrees of freedom, totaling $n \cdot k$.

We can introduce continuity requirements across knot points into Definition B.1. The highest order of continuity that can be imposed is $k-1$ (first order of continuity is continuity in displacement; second, continuity in slope; third, continuity in curvature, and so forth). The reason is rooted in dimensions arithmetic (of counting degrees of freedom); if we demand k degrees of continuity across knot points, then we will get a single continuous polynomial of order k, which is a little too tight a constraint for $n > k$. For $k-1$ orders of continuity across each knot point, we impose only $(n-1) \cdot (k-1)$ constraints over the PP $P(t)$, which leaves us with

$$n \cdot k - (n-1) \cdot (k-1) = n \cdot k - n \cdot k + k + n - 1 \tag{B.4}$$
$$= n+k-1 \text{ degrees of freedom.}$$

In an interpolation problem, we have $n+1$ points p_i, for $i = 0, \ldots, n$, and the problem is to find a PP $P(t)$ such that $P(t_i) = p_i$ for all i. These points impose $n+1$ constraints into the definition of $P(t)$, but by Eq. B.4 we need $k-2$ more constraints to define it uniquely. These additional constraints are termed *boundary conditions* and are imposed arbitrarily on both ends of the interpolation interval.

Continuity constraints are introduced into the definition of $P(t)$ by the vector $A = (a_1, \ldots, a_{n-1})$, where a_i is the number of degrees of continuities required across the internal knot point t_i. The space of all PP-s on the knot sequence T with continuity constraints A is denoted $P_{k,T,A}$. For this space,

$$Dim(P_{k,T,A}) = n \cdot k - \sum_{i=1}^{n-1} a_i. \tag{B.5}$$

B.2.1 Basis Functions

The set of basis function for the space $P_{k,T,A}$, with maximum continuity across internal knot points, i.e., where

$$A = \Big[(k-1), (k-1), \ldots, (k-1)\Big], \tag{B.6}$$

is defined via a set of $n+k-1$ functionals, $\Phi_{i,k}$ (see [DeBoor, 1979]), and a set of functions: $B_{i,k}(t)$ such that the functionals are independent of each other, and

$$\Phi_j(B_{i,k}) = \Delta_{i,j}$$
$$where \quad \Delta_{i,j} = 1 \;\; iff \;\; i=j. \tag{B.7}$$

(i.e., the "delta of Kroneker")

This relation ensures that the functions $B_{i,k}(t)$ are independent. They are defined in the space $P_{k,T,A}$ whose dimension (for A as in Eq. B.6) is $n \cdot k - (n-1) \cdot (k-1) = n+k-1$, exactly as many such functions as there are; therefore, the $B_{i,k}(t)$ are basis functions of this space. That is, if $F(t)$ belongs to this space, then

$$F(t) = \sum_{i=1-k}^{n-1} [\Phi_{i,k}(F) \cdot B_{i,k}(t)]. \tag{B.8}$$

The $\Phi_{i,k}(F)$-s are the *coefficients* for the representation of $F(t)$ in this space of piece-wise polynomials. If $F(t)$ is not in this space, we talk about an approximation, $F'(t)$ for $F(t)$, which is a PP. In general, we will refer to these coefficients as the n-ary vector $\vec{V}$.

We shall not present the definition of $\Phi_{i,k}$; it can be found in [DeBoor, 1979]. Rather, we shall look at a recursive definition that DeBoor, [1972] introduced for the basis functions, $B_{i,k}(t)$

$$B_{i,k}(t) = B_{i,k-1}(t) \cdot \left[\frac{t-t_i}{t_{i+k-1}-t_i} \right] + B_{i+1,k-1}(t) \cdot \left[\frac{t_{i+k}-t}{t_{i+k}-t_{i+1}} \right]; \tag{B.9}$$

$$for \quad t_i \leqslant t < t_{i+k}.$$

Note that this definition takes into account the distance between knot points. This recursive definition for the basis functions was proven correct by DeBoor [1979] based on "divided differences," and will not be repeated here. Note also that a basis function of order k is defined as a *convex combination* of basis functions of order $(k - 1)$. The functions $B_{i,1}$ are shown in Figure B.2. The basis functions $B_{i,1}$ have these properties:

1. Nonnegative;

2. Limited support: positive values inside *one* segment only; and

3. The sum of $B_{i,1}$ (all i) is 1.

Figure B.2.   The basis functions: $B_{i,1} \cdot B_{i,1}(t) = 1$ for $t_1 < t \le t_{i+1}$; 0 otherwise.

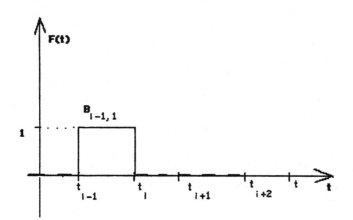

An example of a basis function for $k = 3$ is given in Figure B.3. By the properties of basis functions of order 1 and Eq. B.9, we have the following properties for B-spline functions of any order:

1. $B_{i,k}$ is nonzero on k segments only, the interval $[t_i, t_{i+k}]$ (limited support);

2. It is nonnegative; and

3. $\sum_{i=1}^{n} B_{i,k}(t) = 1.$ (B.10)

Figure B.3.   The basis functions; $B_{i,3}$.

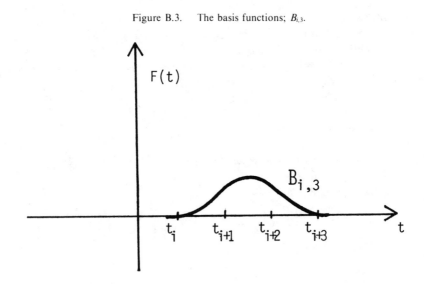

By these and Eq. B.8 it turns out that, to calculate the value of $F(t)$ at any point t, we need only to take into account k elements in the summation of Eq. B.8.

$$P(t) = \sum_{j=i-k+1}^{i} [\Phi_{j,k}(F) \cdot B_{j,k}(t)]$$

for $t \in [i,\ i+1]$.

(B.11)

This property of locality contributes also to computational stability; an error in any of the coefficients $\Phi_{i,k}(F)$ will influence the values calculated for $F(t)$ only in the open interval: (t_i, t_{i+k}).

B.2.2 Basis Functions for the Space $P_{k,T,A}$ (General A)

The general case of A can be converted to a special case of A as in Eq. B.6 by building another set of knot points, X, in which each of the knot points t_i is repeated q_i times, given that the corresponding a_i is $k - 1 - q_i$,

$$\vec{X} = (x_0, \dots, x_m) ,$$

(B.12)

where $m = k + k + \sum_{i=1}^{n-1} (k - a_i)$.

Figure B.4 is an example of how the new knot sequence is defined for $\vec{A} = (1, 2, 2, 3, 0, 1,...)$.

Figure B.4   Definition of the new knot sequence X from T, $A = (...,1,2,2,3,0,1,...)$, and $k = 4$.

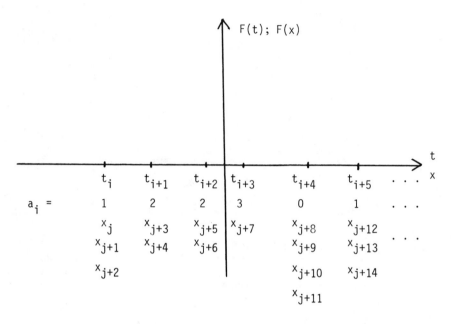

The basis functions for the space $P_{k,x}$ can be defined recursively by Eq. B.9. Some of the segments are of length 0 (null segment) because some of the points in $\vec{X}$ are the same (repeated knot points or coalescing knot points) and will cause discontinuities at knot points. If a_i is $k - 1 - q_i$, i.e., smaller than $k - 1$ by q_i units, then the continuity at knot point t_i will be degraded by q_i degrees, caused by repeating t_i, $1 + q_i$ times in the sequence $\vec{X}$. Figure B.5 demonstrates what happens to those basis functions that have a null segment in their support.

B.2.3 Uniform B-splines

When the t_i-s are equally spaced, we get uniform basis functions in the sense that all have the same *shape*, i.e., equal within parameter translation, and we can calculate one of them once and for all. Each basis function is in the space of piece-wise polynomials and therefore is, by itself, made of pieces. For a given k in the uniform case, we need to find only k polynomials and, by appropriate parameter translations, evaluate the interpolant of $F(t)$ over each of the intervals $[t_i, t_{i+1}]$.

Figure B.6A is a plot of the four pieces of a uniform cubic B-spline ($k = 4$), and Figure B.6B is a plot of the four different pieces of the four different basis functions which have the i-th segment under their support. (The basis functions

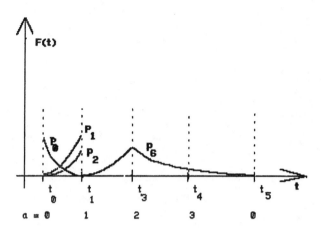

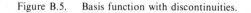

Figure B.6. A) A uniform cubic B-spline; B) The four *different* pieces of the four basis functions that have *i*-th segment under their support; and C) The normalized (for *t* between 0 and 1) cubic polynomials that are the four basic pieces (in B) of the unified basis function (in A).

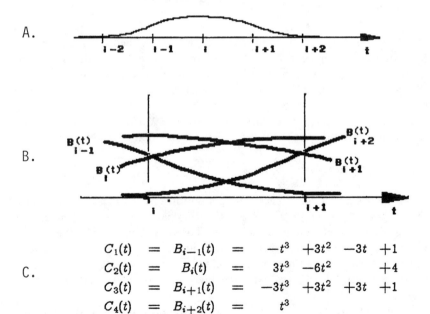

$$C_1(t) = B_{i-1}(t) = -t^3 + 3t^2 - 3t + 1$$
$$C_2(t) = B_i(t) = 3t^3 - 6t^2 + 4$$
$$C_3(t) = B_{i+1}(t) = -3t^3 + 3t^2 + 3t + 1$$
$$C_4(t) = B_{i+2}(t) = t^3$$

are annotated according to the discussion in the next section). Figure B.6C is the analytic definition of the appropriate cubic polynomials.

B.3 Curve Interpolation and Approximation

Here we are interested in curve interpolation in two, or three, dimensions through a list of points. Figure B.7 is an example of such a case. The vector representation of the curve is separated into two functions, $X(t)$ and $Y(t)$. Each of these functions is a piece-wise polynomial of t. For three dimensions, there will be three functions, $X(t)$, $Y(t)$, and $Z(t)$, and so forth.

Riesenfeld [1973] has shown that it does not make a significant difference whether components of a parameterized curve are interpolated by uniform B-splines or nonuniform B-splines, when one judges by the actual appearance of a curve. As shown in Section B.2.3, the uniform approach simplifies matters by letting one deal with only k polynomials of degree k.

The most popular piece-wise polynomial interpolation scheme occurs when $k = 4$ for cubic pieces. Therefore, we hereafter eliminate the index k in formulae. Given the set of interpolation points p_i for $i = 1, \ldots, n$ the interpolant $P(t)$ is a vector-valued piecewise polynomial of the parameter t. This parameter changes uniformly between data points.*

The parameter t can be normalized so that $P(i) = p_i$, i.e., t assumes integer values at data points

$$T = (t_1, \ldots, t_n) = (1, 2, \ldots, n).$$

Each *piece* of $P(t)$ is a cubic polynomial. Globally, $P(t)$ has three orders of continuity across data points (i.e., up to continuity of second-derivative, the curvature). Formally (Formula B.8), $P(t)$ is defined as

$$P(t) = \sum_{i=0}^{n+1} [V_i \cdot B_i(t)] \tag{B.13}$$

or, more precisely, by Eq. B.11 and the above note, for $t\epsilon[i, i+1)$ we have only four nonzero elements in that summation, so that

$$P(t) = \sum_{j=i-1}^{i+2} [V_j \cdot B_j(t)].$$

---

*NOTE

We use a slightly different indexing than in the previous section, ranging from 1 to n, and not from 0 to n, as there. We also change the indexing of basis functions by right-shifting them by 2, so that we have $n+2$ basis functions $B_0, \ldots, B_{n+1}$. This arrangement will provide us with nicely formatted formulae.

The V_i are *coefficients* and serve for the representation of the curve $P(t)$ as a PP. Because they are dual to the set of points P_i, they can be derived from each other.*

The basis functions $B_i(t)$ were presented in Figure B.6, with their four pieces. Each piece in that figure is a polynomial over $t\epsilon[0, 1)$. In the current indexing convention, the basis function $B_i(t)$ will be nonzero only for $t\epsilon[i -2, i + 2)$.

On a given segment $(i, i+1)$ there are only four basis functions that are nonzero, namely: $B_{i-1}(t)$, $B_i(t)$, $B_{i+1}(t)$, and $B_{i+2}(t)$, where only the m-th piece of the $B_{i+2-m}(t)$ is over that segment, for $m = 1,2,3,4$. All the m-th pieces of basis functions are the same (within parameter translation), so we denote the m-th piece as $C_m(t)$ for $0\le t<1$. These cubic polynomials are defined in Figure B.6B, and are termed *basic polynomials*.

To calculate $P(t)$, if t is in the segment $(i, i + 1)$, then

$$P(t) = V_{i-1} \cdot C_4(t-i) + V_i \cdot C_3(t-i)$$
$$+ V_{i+1} \cdot C_2(t-i) + V_{i+2} \cdot C_1(t-i). \qquad \text{(B.15)}$$

Or in matrix notation, using the polynomials $C_m(t)$ defined in Figure B.6B,

$$P_i(t) = [t'^3 \ t'^2 \ t' \ 1] \cdot [C] \cdot$$
$$[V_{i-1} \ V_i \ V_{i+1} \ V_{i+2}]^T \qquad \text{(B.16)}$$
$$t \ \epsilon \ [i, \ i+1], \ \text{and} \ t' = t-i ,$$

---

*NOTE

The number of elements in the summation in Eq. B.13 fits well with Formula B.4; with $k = 4$ and only $(n - 1)$ segments, the dimension of the piece-wise polynomial space is $(n - 1) + 4 - 1 = n + 2$, so we need exactly $n + 2$ coefficients and $n + 2$ basis functions. The interpolation problem is stated with only n interpolation points, so that the extra two coefficients will be determined according to *boundary conditions*. For example, if we want the curvature at the endpoints, $t = 1$ and $t = n$, to be 0, we will require that

$$V_1 = (V_0 + V_2)/2$$
$$V_n = (V_{n-1} + V_{n+1})/2. \qquad \text{(B.14)}$$

which add the two additional needed constraints to uniquely define the PP interpolant.

where $[C]$ is the matrix $\frac{1}{6} \cdot$ $\begin{bmatrix} -1 & 3 & -3 & 1 \\ 3 & -6 & 3 & 0 \\ -3 & 0 & 3 & 0 \\ 1 & 4 & 1 & 0 \end{bmatrix}$

where the elements of the i-th column in the matrix $[C]$ are the coefficients of the cubic polynomial $C_i(t)$, ($i = 1,2,3,4$).

B.3.1 The Conversion Problem

Problem: Given the set of points P_i, how can you determine the PP representation of the interpolant $P(t)$ (such that $P(i) = P_i$), i.e., find the coefficients V_i, and vice versa?

By Eq. B.16, for the i-th piece when $t = i$, then $t' = 0$, and

$$P_i = P(i) = \frac{1}{6} \cdot [0\ 0\ 0\ 1] \cdot [C] \cdot [V_{i-1} \ \cdots \ V_{i+2}]^T$$

$$= \frac{1}{6} \cdot [1\ 4\ 1\ 0] \cdot [V_{i-1} \ \cdots \ V_{i+2}]^T \qquad (B.17)$$

$$= \frac{1}{6} \cdot (V_{i-1} + 4 \cdot V_i + V_{i+1}).$$

When $t = n$, we interpolate the segment $[n - 1, n]$ which for Eq. B.15 means $i = n - 1$, and $t' = 1$:

$$P_n = P(n) = \frac{1}{6} \cdot [1\ 1\ 1\ 1] \cdot [C] \cdot [V_{n-2} \ \cdots \ V_{n+1}]^T$$

$$= \frac{1}{6} \cdot [0\ 1\ 4\ 1] \cdot [V_{n-2} \ \cdots \ V_{n+1}]^T \qquad (B.18)$$

$$= \frac{1}{6} \cdot (V_{n-1} + 4 \cdot V_n + V_{n+1}).$$

Eqs. B.17, B.18 and the boundary conditions in Eq. B.14 provide $n + 2$ equations for the conversion problem:

$$\vec{P} = [D] \cdot \vec{V}$$

where $[D] = \frac{1}{6} \cdot$ $\begin{bmatrix} 6 & & & & & \\ 1 & 4 & 1 & & & \\ & 1 & 4 & 1 & & \\ & & \cdots & & & \\ & & & \cdots & & \\ & & & 1 & 4 & 1 \\ & & & & & 6 \end{bmatrix}$ $\qquad (B.19)$

When interpolating a curve we have to solve for the coefficients for each of the components of the parametric curve representation, i.e., for $X(t)$ and for $Y(t)$; thus by Eq. B.19 we find

$$\vec{V}, \text{ based on } \vec{X} = [X_1, X_2, \cdots X_n]$$

and

$$\vec{U}, \text{ based on } \vec{Y} = [Y_1, Y_2, \cdots Y_n].$$

(B.20)

The matrix in Eq. B.19 is strictly positive and dominantly diagonal, which makes an iterative solution (e.g., Gauss-Seidel) very attractive [Yamaguchi, 1978].

When dealing with closed curves (e.g., Figure B.7), some different boundary conditions than those of Eq. B.14 are needed. When interpolating a closed curve with $n-1$ interpolation points, there are also $n-1$ enclosed segments between them. To fit this situation into the general case of interpolation, we assume that we have n interpolation points, of which the two endpoints are the same, i.e., $P_n = P_1$. For such closed curves, the natural boundary condition is to require the same smoothness across the "meshed" endpoints that there is across any internal point, so that the new boundary conditions are

$$V_{n+1} = V_1$$
$$V_0 = V_{n-1}.$$

(B.21)

The conversion problem will now be (based on Eqs. B.17, B.18, and B.21),

$$\vec{P} = [D_c] \cdot \vec{V}$$

where $[D_c] = \dfrac{1}{6} \cdot \begin{bmatrix} 1 & 4 & & & & & & 1 \\ 1 & 4 & 1 & & & & & \\ & 1 & 4 & 1 & & & & \\ & & \cdots & & & & & \\ & & & \cdots & & & & \\ & & & & 1 & 4 & 1 & \\ & & & & & 1 & 4 & 1 \\ 1 & & & & & & 1 & 4 \end{bmatrix}$

(B.22)

The matrix $[D_c]$ is also strictly positive and diagonal dominant for a stable solution to the conversion problem.

B.3.2 The Variation Diminishing Property

It turns out that the V_i-s are very close to the P_i-s, so that the set of points V_i mimics the interpolant $P(t)$. When viewing curve interpolation, (i.e., Eq. B.20),

Figure B.7.   A 2-D curve interpolated through a list of points. Its vector representation on the right are two functions (for X and Y) of a single parameter t.

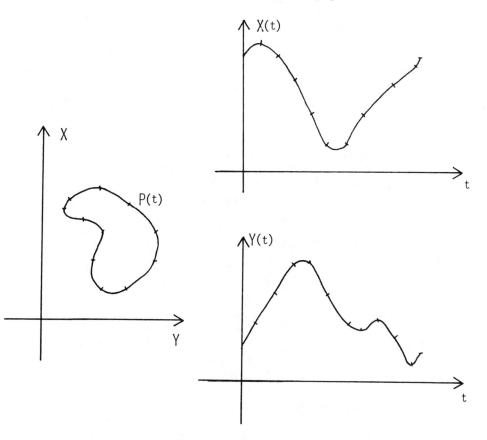

the polyline through the points $[V_i, U_i]$ mimics the curve $[X(t), Y(t)]$ (Figure B.8C). In the general case (see Section B.2.3), the indices of $B_{i,k}$ and P_i were chosen so that $B_{i,k}$ spans the interval $[t_i, t_{i+k}]$ so that the $n + k - 2$ basis functions for the knot sequence $(t_1, \ldots, t_n)$ were

$$B_{2-k,k}(t), B_{3-k,k}(t), \ldots, B_{n-1,k}(t)$$

with coefficients

$$V_{2-k}, \ldots, V_{n-1},$$

and for $k = 4$, it is

$$V_{-2}, V_{-1}, V_0, \ldots, V_{n-1}.$$

Theorem B.1 variation diminishing [Schoenberg]: In uniform B-splines the points $P(i)$ and V_j are very close to each other when j and i are related via

$$j = \frac{(i+1)+(i+2)+ \cdots +(i+k-1)}{k-1}$$

and for $k = 4$

$$j = \frac{(i+1)+(i+2)+(i+3)}{3} = i+2$$

By this theorem, $V_{i+2} \approx P_i$, so that by shifting the indices of the B_i-s and the V_i-s by 2 to the right, we get the enumeration as in Section B.3, namely $B_0, \dots, B_{n+1}$, $V_0, \dots, V_{n+1}$, and have the property that V_i is closest to P_i. At the same time, the interpolation in the i-th segment ($[i,i + 1]$) is a "blend" of the four basic polynomials, $C_m(t)$, by the four "enclosing" coefficients $V_{i-1}, \dots, V_{i+2}$. This property of cubic uniform B-splines is mostly attractive to computer graphics and CAD/CAM. It was primarily promoted by Riesenfeld [1973] in his Ph.D. thesis, and has produced attractive results [Wu, 1977]. In these applications, the interpolation points P_i were taken as the coefficients V_i, termed also "control- points" (they control the curve shape). When linearly interpolating the control-points, we get what is called the "guiding polygon" for closed curves, or a "guiding polyline" for open curves. In such cases, the conversion problem is eliminated, but the resulting curve is only an *approximation* to the given control-points. The new P_i-s that correspond to the control-points are obtained (if one is interested in them) by direct substitutions in Eqs. B.17 and B.18.

The variation diminishing property means that, when one passes a straight line through the polyline (linear interpolation between points) defined by the points V_i, the line will intersect the polyline at least as many times as it will intersect the polyline defined by the points P_i. Moreover, this straight line will not intersect the curve $P(t)$ more times. Figure B.8B demonstrates that point.

The three most appreciated properties of variation diminishing splines are (for cubic splines) the following:

1. The approximated smooth curve lies in the convex hull of the guiding polygon, or more precisely, each segment of the interpolant lies in the convex-hull of the polyline defined by the corresponding four control-points (used to interpolate it) (Figure B.8A).

2. Locality is expressed by limiting the effect on the curve shape when a single control-point is moved (cf. Figure B.8B) to only four segments of the curve. That is, if we move V_i, then only the segment between P_{i-1} and P_{i+2} is affected ($i = 1, \dots, n-1$).

Figure B.8.   A) The approximated curve is in the convex hull of the guiding polygon; B) Locality is demonstrated: when a control-point V_i is moved, only a short portion (of 4 segments) of the curve is changed; and C) Drawing a face profile with open B-spline curve, guided by an "open" polygon (or a polyline). (B and C are taken from "An Interactive Computer Graphics Approach to Surface Representation" by Sheng-Chuan Wu, John F. Abel, and Donald P. Greenberg, *Communications of the ACM* 20(10), pp. 703-712 (October, 1977),

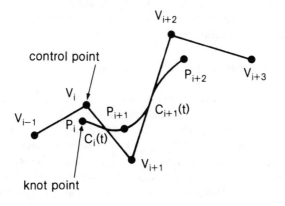

$P_i - P_{i+1}$ is in the quadruple $V_{i-1} - V_{i+2}$

$P_{i+1} - P_{i+2}$ is in the quadruple $V_i - V_{i+3}$

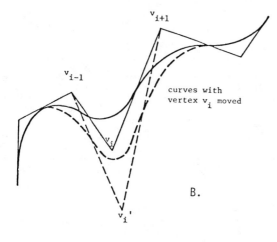

curves with vertex v_i moved

B.

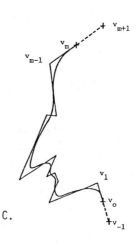

C.

3. Given the V_i-s, a curve can be efficiently approximated for rapid graphic rendition of shapes (see in particular [Wu, 1977]).

B.4 Manipulating Uniform Cubic B-Splines

Given the PP spline definition of a curve, we would like to find what can be done with it when geometry of the defined shape is concerned. Geometric properties of concern are the intersection of a spline curve with other curves, calculation of the enclosed area between a planar spline curve and the origin, and the curve slope and curvature at an arbitrary point.

B.4.1 Intersection with Other Curves

Eq. B.16 defines a uniform cubic B-spline curve in a constructive way, i.e., implicitly. As the parameter t changes incrementally, we determine points that belong to the curve, $\vec{P}(t)$. Let's say that we are given the equation for another curve, $\vec{C}$, explicitly, i.e., for any point $\vec{p}$ we can *test* whether it is on the curve $\vec{C}$ or not by substitution, to try how accurately it solves the given equation. Our problem is to determine whether (and for what value of t) the curve $\vec{C}$ intersects the given spline curve $\vec{P}(t)$. We can substitute $\vec{P}(t)$ in the equation for $\vec{C}$ to obtain an equation of the unknown t, which we can solve in any desired way. A relatively easy case is that in which $\vec{C}$ is a straight line. We shall demonstrate the problem of finding the intersections, if any, of the straight line $\vec{L}$ and the uniform cubic B-spline $\vec{P}(t)$ by the following example.

Example: We rewrite Eq. B.16:

$$\vec{P}_i(t) = [T] \cdot [C] \cdot [V]_i{}^T ,\qquad\qquad (B.16A)$$

where $[T] = [t^3\ t^2\ t\ 1]$

$$[V]_i = \begin{bmatrix} X_{i-1} & X_i & X_{i+1} & X_{i+2} \\ Y_{i-1} & Y_i & Y_{i+1} & Y_{i+2} \end{bmatrix}$$

The general equation of a straight line is

$$\vec{p} \cdot [L]^T = c ,\qquad\qquad (B.23)$$

where

p is a point (i.e., $[x,y]$ in 2-D)
$[L]$ is a constant vector (i.e., $[a,b]$ in 2-D)
c is a constant scalar.
       (i.e., in 2-D we have the equation $a \cdot x \times b \cdot y = c$)

To find the intersection point we substitute Eq. B.16A in Eq. B.23 for p, and get

$$[T] \cdot [C] \cdot [V]_i^T \cdot [L]^T = c. \tag{B.24}$$

The problem is not solved yet because we have two unknowns: t and i. According to our formalism, t can range only from 0 to 1, per i, but Eq. B.24 may have solutions of "illegal" t. Therefore, we have to solve that equation for all $i = 1, \ldots, n-1$ and let t vary appropriately in each of these pieces of $P(t)$ so that there will be no overlapping. The following algorithm is proposed for this problem:

Algorithm B.1:

comment Algorithm for finding the points of intersection for the uniform cubic B-spline curve $\vec{P}(t)$ and a straight line;

> *for* i:= 1 *step* 1 *until* $n-1$ *do*
> > *begin*
> > > solve $[T] \cdot [C] \cdot [V]_i^T \cdot [L]^T = c$ for t;
> > >
> > > assume t_j $(j = 1,2,3)$ are the solutions;
> > >
> > > *for* j:= 1 *step* 1 *until* 3 *do*
> > > > *begin*
> > > > > *if* t_j is real *and* $(0 < t_j \leqslant 1)$ *then*
> > > > > > (t_j, i) is a solution;
> > > > *end;*
> > *end;*

Demonstration:

If $[V_i] = \begin{bmatrix} 0 & 0 & 1 & 2 \\ 2 & 1 & 0 & 1 \end{bmatrix}$

and
$[L] = [1 \; -1]$

$c = 0$

then Eq. B.24 becomes

$$[t^3 \; t^2 \; t \; 1] \cdot [C] \cdot \begin{bmatrix} 0 & 2 \\ 0 & 1 \\ 1 & 0 \\ 2 & 0 \end{bmatrix} \cdot \begin{bmatrix} 1 \\ -1 \end{bmatrix} = 0,$$

$$[t^3 \; t^2 \; t \; 1] \cdot [C] \cdot [-6 \; -3 \; 1 \; 2]^T = 0,$$

which results in

$$\frac{1}{6} \cdot (-2t^3 + 3t^2 + 9t - 5) = 0,$$

for which the solutions are

$$t_1 = -1.79128784$$

$$t_2 = -2.79128784$$

$$t_3 = 0.5.$$

Thus, the point of intersection is for $t = t_3 = 0.5 \rightarrow p = [0.5208, 0.5208]$. The situation is plotted in Figure B.9.

Figure B.9.   Demonstrating the intersection of a B-spline curve by a straight line.

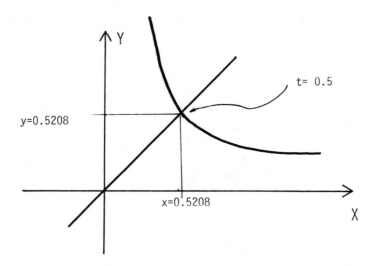

B.4.2 Tangents and Curvatures

The parametric curve of Eq. B.1 $\vec{C}(t) = [X(t), Y(t)]$ has at each point t a tangent vector if the curve is continuous in its derivatives at this point (since each piece of a PP is continuous, discontinuities may occur only at knot points).

The derivative is

$$\frac{\partial \vec{V}(t)}{\partial t} = \left[\frac{\partial X(t)}{\partial t}, \frac{\partial Y(t)}{\partial t} \right] \tag{B.25}$$

And by Eq. B.16, we get for each component of the tangent vector

$$\frac{\partial \vec{X}(t)}{\partial t} = [3t^2 \; 2t \; 1] \cdot [C']$$

$$\cdot [X_{i-1} \; X_i \; X_{i+1} \; X_{i+2}]^T, \qquad (B.26)$$

where $[C']$ is a matrix composed of the first three rows of $[C]$ in Eq. B.16.

The second derivative is a vector normal to the curve. (For 3-D curves, this can be interpreted as the vector orthogonal to the tangent vector that lies in the plane of an infinitesimal portion of the curve in the neighborhood of the point. If the curve has curvature 0 at this point, i.e., it is a straight line, then the curvature direction is singular):

$$\frac{\partial^2 \vec{V}(t)}{\partial V^2} = \left[\frac{\partial^2 X(t)}{\partial X^2}, \; \frac{\partial^2 Y(t)}{\partial Y^2} \right]. \qquad (B.27)$$

The formula for each of the components in the above vector is derived from Eq. B.16 in the same manner as that for Eq. B.26:

$$\frac{\partial^2 \vec{V}(t)}{\partial t^2} = [6t^2 \; 2] \cdot [C'']$$

$$\cdot [X_{i-1} \; X_i \; X_{i+1} \; X_{i+2}]^T, \qquad (B.28)$$

where $[C'']$ is made of the first two rows of $[C]$ in Eq. B.16.

B.4.3 Area Enclosed by a 2-D B-spline Curve

It is interesting to find the area enclosed by a closed B-spline curve, and its centroid. The area and its centroid are also interesting for *open* curves (cf. Figure B.10), for which a closed curve is a special case. For planar parametric curves (see Figure B.10) the area enclosed by some arc, in which the parameter t ranges between t_0 and t_1, the origin, and the two rays from the origin to the points $\vec{p}(t_0)$ and $\vec{p}(t_1)$ is given by

$$A(X,Y,t_0,t_1) = \int_{t_0}^{t_1} \frac{\partial A(t)}{\partial t} \; dt$$

$$= \int_{t_0}^{t_1} \left[X(t) \frac{\partial Y(t)}{\partial t} - Y(t) \frac{\partial X(t)}{\partial t} \right] dt \qquad (B.29)$$

$$= [A_{x,y} + A_{y,x}](X,Y,t_0,t_1).$$

Figure B.10. The area "enclosed" by a parametric arc and the origin.

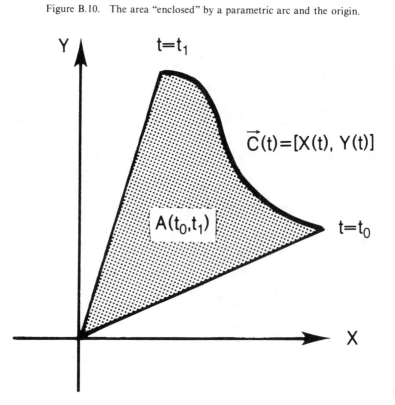

When the curve is a B-spline, we have to integrate in pieces. If t_0 is in the j-th piece and t_1 is in the k-th piece, let's define

$$L = t_0 - j,$$
$$H = k + 1 - t_1 \tag{B.30}$$

and

$$A^i(L) = A(X_i, Y_i, O, L)$$
$$\text{where} \quad 0 < L \leqslant 1$$

and $X_i(t)$, $Y_i(t)$ correspond to the i-th pieces of the B-spline interpolants for $X(t)$ and $Y(t)$, respectively. Let's also define $A^i = A^i(1)$, which is the area enclosed by the i-th segment. Now the area for the B-spline will be

$$A(t_0, t_1) = \sum_{i=j}^{k-1} (A^i) + A^k(H) - A^j(L). \tag{B.31}$$

The spline curve is represented as in Eq. B.16A: the X element of $[V]_i$ is $[V_x]_i$ and the Y element is $[V_y]_i$. By Section B.4.2, the derivatives are

$$\frac{\partial X_i(t)}{\partial t} = [3t^2 \ 2t \ 1 \ 0] \cdot [C] \cdot [V_x]_i^T. \tag{B.32}$$

For simplicity we avoid the subscript i in further formulations and denote the derivative as $dX(t)$, which is understood as part of the calculation for $A^i(L)$.

Our purpose is to simplify the contents of the integral in Eq. B.29 while retaining the convenient matrix representation in Eq. B.32.

$$X(t) \cdot \frac{\partial Y(t)}{\partial t} =$$

$$= [t^3 \ t^2 \ t \ 1] \cdot [C] \cdot [V_x]^T \cdot [3t^3 \ 2t \ 1 \ 0] \cdot [C] \cdot [V_y]^T$$

$$= [V_x] \cdot [C]^T \cdot [t^3 \ t^2 \ t \ 1]^T \cdot [3t^2 \ 2t \ 1 \ 0] \cdot [C] \cdot [V_y]^T \tag{B.33}$$

$$= [V_x] \cdot [C]^T \cdot [M_1](t) \cdot [C] \cdot [V_y]^T$$

$$\text{where} \quad [M_1](t) = \begin{vmatrix} 3t^5 & 2t^4 & t^3 & 0 \\ 3t^4 & 2t^3 & t^2 & 0 \\ 3t^3 & 2t^2 & t & 0 \\ 3t^2 & 2t & 1 & 0 \end{vmatrix}$$

Since only $[M_1]$ contains the variable t, we can take everything else out of the integral expression or try to calculate the integral for $[M_1]$ only:

$$[N](L) = \int_0^L [M_1](t) \, dt =$$

$$= \begin{vmatrix} L^6/2 & 2L^5/5 & L^4/4 & 0 \\ 3L^5/5 & L^4/2 & L^3/3 & 0 \\ 3L^4/4 & 2L^3/3 & L^2/2 & 0 \\ L^3 & L^2 & L & 0 \end{vmatrix} \tag{B.34A}$$

and when $L = 1$,

$$[Q] = [N](1) = \int_0^1 [M_1](t) \, dt =$$

$$= \begin{vmatrix} 1/2 & 2/5 & 1/4 & 0 \\ 3/5 & 1/2 & 1/3 & 0 \\ 3/4 & 2/3 & 1/2 & 0 \\ 1 & 1 & 1 & 0 \end{vmatrix} \tag{B.34B}$$

Going back to Eq. B.29,

$$A^i = [V_x] \cdot [C]^T \cdot [Q] \cdot [C] \cdot [V_y]^T - [V_y] \cdot [C]^T \cdot [Q] \cdot [C] \cdot [V_x]^T,$$
$$= [V_x] \cdot [C]^T \cdot ([Q] - [Q]^T) \cdot [C] \cdot [V_y]^T$$
$$= [V_x] \cdot [M] \cdot [V_y]^T,$$

where $[M] = [C]^T \cdot ([Q] - [Q]^T) \cdot [C] =$ (B.35A)

$$= \begin{bmatrix} 0 & 31/10 & 14/5 & 1/10 \\ -31/10 & 0 & 183/10 & 14/5 \\ -14/5 & -183/10 & 0 & 31/10 \\ -1/10 & -14/5 & -31/10 & 0 \end{bmatrix}$$

If we use $[N]$ (L) in Eq. B.35A, we get in the formula for $A^i(L)$ a matrix that corresponds to $[M]$, which is so large that we show only the matrix $[N](L) - [N]^T(L)$:

$$[N](L) - [N]^T(L) =$$

$$= \begin{bmatrix} 0 & -L^5/5 & -L^4/2 & -L^3 \\ L^5/5 & 0 & -L^3/3 & -L^2 \\ L^4/2 & L^3/3 & 0 & -L \\ L^3 & L^2 & L & 0 \end{bmatrix} \quad\quad\quad (B.35B)$$

Another interesting formula is for the center of gravity, or *centroid* $[X_c, Y_c]$, *which for* X_c is

$$X_c = \frac{1}{3A} \int_0^1 \left[x_i(t)^2 \frac{\partial}{\partial t} y_i(t) - x_i(t) \cdot y_i(t) \cdot \frac{\partial}{\partial t} x_i(t) \right] dt \quad\quad (B.36)$$

where A is the total area enclosed. A similar formula will also work for Y_c. This formula can be expressed in the same compact way as it was done for the area, though it is much more complex and will not be presented here.

Appendix C

Example: Model Representation

This appendix lists the internal model structure explained in Chapter 4, and in references to Figure 4.1.

The model is internally represented as a hierarchical associative network. For the purpose of this listing the network is traversed, beginning with an organ node, following all its associations, and repeating this process on all new encountered nodes. Each recovered association is printed as

<ATTRIBUTE> : <value>

where <value> may be another item with associations or a set of such items to be further traversed or a data structure that is printed right away. Whenever an item is traced, its PNAME is printed, but if it has no PNAME, then some unique characterizing string will issue instead. Only the left kidney is pursued in detail.

```
Attributes of Left Kidney:
————————————————————
Organ modifier:    Kidney Modifier
Organ expert:      Kidney organ expert
Organ center:      real array[1:3]
   [ 80.0    ] [ 70.0    ] [-70.0    ]

Organ center tolerance:    real array[1:3]
   [ 15.0    ] [ 15.0    ] [ 15.0    ]

Organ size:      real array[1:3]
   [ 40.0    ] [ 40.0    ] [ 80.0    ]

Organ size tolerance:    real array[1:3]
   [ 15.0    ] [ 15.0    ] [ 25.0    ]

Tissue type:        520
Surrounding tissue:      455
Organ descriptor: 'LKDNY'
Organ shape:    set of:
————————————————
ITEM!0270:   :
   Spline name:      'LKDNY1'
   Spline color:     2
   Spline values:    real array[1:4,1:2]
   ⎡-6.00    ⎤ ⎡ .000    ⎤
   ⎢ .000    ⎥ ⎢ 6.00    ⎥
   ⎢ 6.00    ⎥ ⎢ .000    ⎥
   ⎣ .000    ⎦ ⎣-6.00    ⎦

   Spline continuity:       '1111'
   X Spline center:  .000
   Y Spline center:  .000
   Z Spline center: -35.0
   Slice Expert:    Kidney slice expert
   Slice center:     real array[1:3]
   [ .000    ] [ .000    ] [-35.0    ]

   Slice values:      real array[1:4,1:2]
   ⎡-6.00    ⎤ ⎡ .000    ⎤
   ⎢ .000    ⎥ ⎢ 6.00    ⎥
   ⎢ 6.00    ⎥ ⎢ .000    ⎥
   ⎣ .000    ⎦ ⎣-6.00    ⎦

   Slice size:      real array[1:2]
   [ 12.0    ] [ 12.0    ]

   Slice instance size:      real array[1:2]
   [ 12.0    ] [ 12.0    ]

   Slice modifier: Kidney slice Modifier
   MatchRtns:        list of:
   ————————————
      Gradient:      :
         ITEM!0119: value type: 8
      Gradient:      :
         ITEM!0119: value type: 8
      Gradient:      :
         ITEM!0119: value type: 8
      Gradient:      :
         ITEM!0119: value type: 8
ITEM!0313:   :
   Spline name:      'LKDNY2'
   Spline color:     2
   Spline values:    real array[1:4,1:2]
   ⎡-10.0    ⎤ ⎡ .000    ⎤
   ⎢ .000    ⎥ ⎢ 10.0    ⎥
   ⎢ 10.0    ⎥ ⎢ .000    ⎥
   ⎣ .000    ⎦ ⎣-10.0    ⎦
```

```
   Spline continuity:       '1111'
   X Spline center:  .000
   Y Spline center:  .000
   Z Spline center: -30.0
   Slice Expert:    Kidney slice expert
   Slice center:     real array[1:3]
   [ .000    ] [ .000    ] [-30.0    ]

   Slice values:      real array[1:4,1:2]
   ⎡-10.0    ⎤ ⎡ .000    ⎤
   ⎢ .000    ⎥ ⎢ 10.0    ⎥
   ⎢ 10.0    ⎥ ⎢ .000    ⎥
   ⎣ .000    ⎦ ⎣-10.0    ⎦

   Slice size:      real array[1:2]
   [ 20.0    ] [ 20.0    ]

   Slice instance size:      real array[1:2]
   [ 20.0    ] [ 20.0    ]

   Slice modifier: Kidney slice Modifier
   MatchRtns:        list of:
   ————————————
      Gradient:      :
         ITEM!0119: value type: 8
      Gradient:      :
         ITEM!0119: value type: 8
      Gradient:      :
         ITEM!0119: value type: 8
      Gradient:      :
         ITEM!0119: value type: 8
ITEM!0279:   :
   Spline name:      'LKDNY3'
   Spline color:     2
   Spline values:    real array[1:4,1:2]
   ⎡-16.0    ⎤ ⎡ .000    ⎤
   ⎢ .000    ⎥ ⎢ 16.0    ⎥
   ⎢ 16.0    ⎥ ⎢ .000    ⎥
   ⎣ .000    ⎦ ⎣-16.0    ⎦

   Spline continuity:       '1111'
   X Spline center:  .000
   Y Spline center:  .000
   Z Spline center: -20.0
   Slice Expert:    Kidney slice expert
   Slice center:     real array[1:3]
   [ .000    ] [ .000    ] [-20.0    ]

   Slice values:      real array[1:4,1:2]
   ⎡-16.0    ⎤ ⎡ .000    ⎤
   ⎢ .000    ⎥ ⎢ 16.0    ⎥
   ⎢ 16.0    ⎥ ⎢ .000    ⎥
   ⎣ .000    ⎦ ⎣-16.0    ⎦

   Slice size:      real array[1:2]
   [ 32.0    ] [ 32.0    ]

   Slice instance size:      real array[1:2]
   [ 32.0    ] [ 32.0    ]

   Slice modifier: Kidney slice Modifier
   MatchRtns:        list of:
   ————————————
      Gradient:      :
         ITEM!0119: value type: 8
      Gradient:      :
         ITEM!0119: value type: 8
      Back Gradient:      :
         ITEM!0119: value type: 8
      Back Gradient:      :
```

```
                ITEM!0119: value type: 8
ITEM!0261:   :
  Spline name:       'LKDNY4'
  Spline color:      2
  Spline values:     real array[1:4,1:2]
     [-20.0  ] [ .000  ]
     [  .000 ] [ 20.0  ]
     [ 20.0  ] [ .000  ]
     [  .000 ] [-20.0  ]

  Spline continuity:       '1111'
  X Spline center:  .000
  Y Spline center:  .000
  Z Spline center: -10.0
  Slice Expert:    Kidney slice expert
  Slice center:      real array[1:3]
     [ .000  ] [ .000  ] [-10.0   ]

  Slice values:      real array[1:4,1:2]
     [-20.0  ] [ .000  ]
     [  .000 ] [ 20.0  ]
     [ 20.0  ] [ .000  ]
     [  .000 ] [-20.0  ]

  Slice size:        real array[1:2]
     [ 40.0  ] [ 40.0  ]

  Slice instance size:     real array[1:2]
     [ 40.0  ] [ 40.0  ]

  Slice modifier:  Kidney slice Modifier
  MatchRtns:         list of:
  ───────────
     Gradient:      :
          ITEM!0119: value type: 8
     DontCare:      :
          ITEM!0119: value type: 8
     Back Gradient:       :
          ITEM!0119: value type: 8
     Back Gradient:       :
          ITEM!0119: value type: 8
ITEM!0322:   :
  Spline name:       'LKDNY5'
  Spline color:      2
  Spline values:     real array[1:4,1:2]
     [-21.0  ] [ .000  ]
     [  .000 ] [ 21.0  ]
     [ 21.0  ] [ .000  ]
     [  .000 ] [-21.0  ]

  Spline continuity:       '1111'
  X Spline center:  .000
  Y Spline center:  .000
  Z Spline center:  .000
  Slice Expert:    Kidney slice expert
  Slice center:      real array[1:3]
     [ .000  ] [ .000  ] [ .000   ]

  Slice values:      real array[1:4,1:2]
     [-21.0  ] [ .000  ]
     [  .000 ] [ 21.0  ]
     [ 21.0  ] [ .000  ]
     [  .000 ] [-21.0  ]

  Slice size:        real array[1:2]
     [ 42.0  ] [ 42.0  ]

  Slice instance size:       real array[1:2]
     [ 42.0  ] [ 42.0  ]
```

```
  Slice modifier:  Kidney slice Modifier
  MatchRtns:         list of:
  ───────────
     Gradient:      :
          ITEM!0119: value type: 8
     DontCare:      :
          ITEM!0119: value type: 8
     Back Gradient:      :
          ITEM!0119: value type: 8
     Back Gradient:      :
          ITEM!0119: value type: 8
ITEM!0220:   :
  Spline name:       'LKDNY6'
  Spline color:      2
  Spline values:     real array[1:4,1:2]
     [-20.0  ] [ .000  ]
     [  .000 ] [ 20.0  ]
     [ 20.0  ] [ .000  ]
     [  .000 ] [-20.0  ]

  Spline continuity:       '1111'
  X Spline center:  .000
  Y Spline center:  .000
  Z Spline center:  10.0
  Slice Expert:    Kidney slice expert
  Slice center:      real array[1:3]
     [ .000  ] [ .000  ] [ 10.0   ]

  Slice values:      real array[1:4,1:2]
     [-20.0  ] [ .000  ]
     [  .000 ] [ 20.0  ]
     [ 20.0  ] [ .000  ]
     [  .000 ] [-20.0  ]

  Slice size:        real array[1:2]
     [ 40.0  ] [ 40.0  ]

  Slice instance size:       real array[1:2]
     [ 40.0  ] [ 40.0  ]

  Slice modifier:  Kidney slice Modifier
  MatchRtns:         list of:
  ───────────
     Gradient:      :
          ITEM!0119: value type: 8
     DontCare:      :
          ITEM!0119: value type: 8
     Back Gradient:      :
          ITEM!0119: value type: 8
     Back Gradient:      :
          ITEM!0119: value type: 8
ITEM!0285:   :
  Spline name:       'LKDNY7'
  Spline color:      2
  Spline values:     real array[1:4,1:2]
     [-16.0  ] [ .000  ]
     [  .000 ] [ 16.0  ]
     [ 16.0  ] [ .000  ]
     [  .000 ] [-16.0  ]

  Spline continuity:       '1111'
  X Spline center:  .000
  Y Spline center:  .000
  Z Spline center:  20.0
  Slice Expert:    Kidney slice expert
  Slice center:      real array[1:3]
     [ .000  ] [ .000  ] [ 20.0   ]

  Slice values:      real array[1:4,1:2]
     [-16.0  ] [ .000  ]
```

```
[ .000  ] [  16.0 ]
[ 16.0  ] [  .000 ]
[ .000  ] [ -16.0 ]
```

Slice size: real array[1:2]
```
[ 32.0 ] [ 32.0 ]
```

Slice instance size: real array[1:2]
```
[ 32.0 ] [ 32.0 ]
```

Slice modifier: Kidney slice Modifier
MatchRtns: list of:

    Gradient: :
        ITEM!0119: value type: 8
    Gradient: :
        ITEM!0119: value type: 8
    Back Gradient: :
        ITEM!0119: value type: 8
    Back Gradient: :
        ITEM!0119: value type: 8
ITEM!0332:   :
  Spline name: 'LKDNY8'
  Spline color: 2
  Spline values: real array[1:4,1:2]
```
[ -10.0 ] [  .000 ]
[  .000 ] [ 10.0  ]
[ 10.0  ] [  .000 ]
[  .000 ] [ -10.0 ]
```

  Spline continuity: '1111'
  X Spline center: .000
  Y Spline center: .000
  Z Spline center: 30.0
  Slice Expert: Kidney slice expert
  Slice center: real array[1:3]
```
[ .000  ] [ .000  ] [ 30.0 ]
```

  Slice values: real array[1:4,1:2]
```
[ -10.0 ] [  .000 ]
[  .000 ] [ 10.0  ]
[ 10.0  ] [  .000 ]
[  .000 ] [ -10.0 ]
```

  Slice size: real array[1:2]
```
[ 20.0 ] [ 20.0 ]
```

  Slice instance size: real array[1:2]
```
[ 20.0 ] [ 20.0 ]
```

  Slice modifier: Kidney slice Modifier
  MatchRtns: list of:

    Gradient: :
        ITEM!0119: value type: 8
    Gradient: :
        ITEM!0119: value type: 8
    Gradient: :
        ITEM!0119: value type: 8
    Gradient: :
        ITEM!0119: value type: 8
ITEM!0289:   :
  Spline name: 'LKDNY9'
  Spline color: 2
  Spline values: real array[1:4,1:2]
```
[ -6.00 ] [  .000 ]
[  .000 ] [ 6.00  ]
[ 6.00  ] [  .000 ]
[  .000 ] [ -6.00 ]
```

Spline continuity: '1111'
X Spline center: .000
Y Spline center: .000
Z Spline center: 35.0
Slice Expert: Kidney slice expert
Slice center: real array[1:3]
```
[ .000  ] [ .000  ] [ 35.0 ]
```

Slice values: real array[1:4,1:2]
```
[ -6.00 ] [  .000 ]
[  .000 ] [ 6.00  ]
[ 6.00  ] [  .000 ]
[  .000 ] [ -6.00 ]
```

Slice size: real array[1:2]
```
[ 12.0 ] [ 12.0 ]
```

Slice instance size: real array[1:2]
```
[ 12.0 ] [ 12.0 ]
```

Slice modifier: Kidney slice Modifier
MatchRtns: list of:

    Gradient: :
        ITEM!0119: value type: 8
    Gradient: :
        ITEM!0119: value type: 8
    Gradient: :
        ITEM!0119: value type: 8
    Gradient: :
        ITEM!0119: value type: 8

Organ tissue tolerance:5
Organ-instance center: real array[1:3]
```
[ 80.0 ] [ 70.0 ] [ -70.0 ]
```

Organ-instance size: real array[1:3]
```
[ 40.0 ] [ 40.0 ] [ 80.0 ]
```

Organ orientation: real array[1:4,1:4]
```
[ 1.00 ] [ .000 ] [ .000 ] [ .000 ]
[ .000 ] [ 1.00 ] [ .000 ] [ .000 ]
[ .000 ] [ .000 ] [ 1.00 ] [ .000 ]
[ .000 ] [ .000 ] [ .000 ] [ 1.00 ]
```

Spinal Column: Neighbour 2

Neighbour 2:   :
  Touching: 0
  Distance: real array[1:3]
```
[ 50.0 ] [ -10.0 ] [ .000 ]
```

  Organ distance tolerance: real array[1:3]
```
[ 10.0 ] [ 10.0 ] [ 10.0 ]
```

Appendix D

Data Acquisition and Representation

D.1 Introduction

Figure D.1 depicts the general data acquisition path. The CT/T CAT-scanner is located at the Radiology department in Strong Memorial Hospital, where a selected scan is archived on a magnetic tape in a General Electric Company designed format. The tape is then mounted on a PDP10 computer, and the archived scan is converted to a 3-D image on a disk. In this appendix we will describe the structure of the 3-D image representation and the conversion process from the General Electric format.

Figure D.1.   Data acquisition.

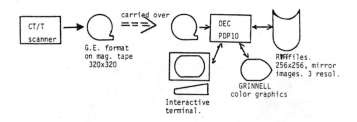

D.2 Format Conversion

A CAT scan is archived on a magnetic tape as a single file. Logically, it consists of several *slices,* each with its own identifying *header,* and the whole set of slices is preceded with an *information header* that contains packing parameters also. Each slice is a 2-D image that compactly represents the reconstructed portion of the image, thus describing an elliptical-shaped (almost circular) image made of a collection of *scan lines* of varying lengths. The information header contains also details of voxel size, patient identification, and scanning conditions and description. The header of each slice contains also the "Zlevel," or the *index* that corresponds to its Z coordinate relative to the body (cf. Figure 3.2A).

The image is converted to a set of RIFF (Raster Image File Format) files [Selfridge, 1979]. Each RIFF file represents a rectangular raster image as a set of *scan lines* of equal lengths. The image parameters specify the number of scan lines, their size, some machine-dependent information about pixel packing, and the pixel scanning order. The RIFF format reflects the assumption that images are obtained by scanning a picture in some order and with some resolution, to produce a stream of digitized pixels. The array of pixel values in each RIFF file are preceded by a *header* that contains the image parameters and (optionally) additional values that are associated with names for convenient storage and retrieval, termed NTV's (for Name-Type-Value triple).

Figure A.1 (Appendix A) is an original CAT slice which is a 320 × 320 image, for which (compatible with radiology conventions) the left side is of the right side of the scanned body. To comply with the coordinate system defined for the body in this work (Figure 3.2A), each slice is *mirror-imaged* before being stored as a RIFF file, as depicted in Figure D.2. From storage limitation reasons, each RIFF file is a window of 256 × 256 pixels from the original image. For each slice, three images are created in three resolutions. Each resolution is defined to have some *resolution factor,* so that the highest resolution is of resolution factor 1, the original resolution. An image of resolution factor n is made by averaging the pixel values of a corresponding $n \times n$ subimage of the original image. The three resolution factors are 1, 4, and 16, shown in Figures D.2 and D.3.

Figure D.2.   A RIFF image of a CAT scan slice is a 256 × 256 window from a mirror image of the original slice.

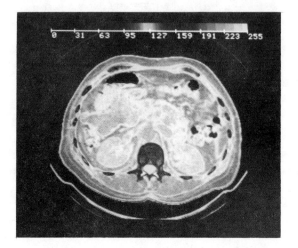

Figure D.3.   Three resolution factors: (Resolution factor 1 is
              shown in Figure D.1.) A) Resolution factor 4; and B)
              Resolution factor 16.

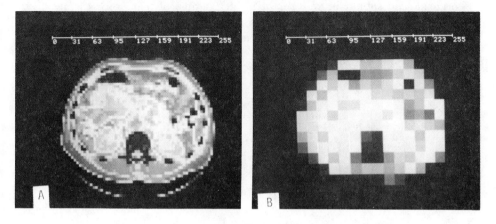

Figure D.4.   A 2-D analogy (with pixels) for the definition of voxel
              "territory" for the various resolution factors. A pixel
              of resolution-factor 1 (a dot) is outlined with thin
              lines, and a pixel of resolution-factor 4 (an x) is
              outlined with saturated lines. The value of point
              $[x_0, y_0]$ is interpolated via the four closest pixels (for
              the case of resolution-factor 4).

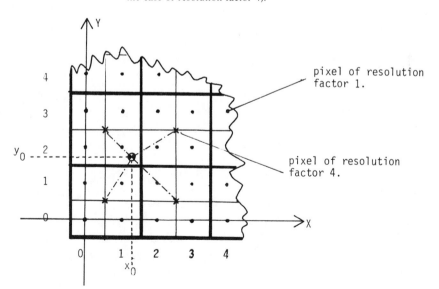

In the header of each RIFF file thus generated, we record the *Zlevel*, the *Resolution*, the *Xsize*, and the *Ysize* parameters for the image. The conversion process is carried out by a program that takes user commands as to how the original scan should be re-formatted. An example of that process is given below, for generating RIFF files as described above. In this listing, the information on all headers of the scan are printed and interpreted. The patient name, however, is abbreviated.

Listing D.1:

Welcome to CT-scans striper program.
Please make sure you are on the
apropriate file on the tape, or
use DEC's "skip" command to do so.
                           Uri Shani

Enter device name [default is '']: in

Enter base disk file name
[default is '']: H

Enter ppn and sfd for files name
[default is '']:

 are you on the ALTO and want a
histogram analysis?[Y or N] n No

Enter Number of resolution levels
[Deafult is:0]=3
 --> 3
Enter resolution factor
[Deafult is:0]=4
 --> 4
Want a scaled down image for ALTOifying
later?[Y or N] n No

Want to invert the scan direction ?
[Y or N] y Yes

12Archived File name: 20642
Patient ID= 1061423
Patient name= J. M., 53
Scan Description:
     LIVER CT SCAN POST ANGIO
Body scan
Contrust agent= POST ANGIO
Position reference= XY
Views per frame= 2
Top view number= 200
Withcontrust agent
DAS type: 16Bits
Number of slices taken= 24
Starting slice number= 1
Last slice number= 24
Incremental between slices= -10
Table index for this current slice= -45
Feet first
Date: date= 07/14/80
Hospital name= SMH ROCH.NY
scan start time= 13:24:54
scan stop time= 13:54:45
pixsiz= 1.100000
ydiam= 35.00000   xdiam= 35.00000
Max pixels per scan line= 318.0000
Information line range= 1 - 320
Want to set a window?[Y or N] y Yes
Enter Scan width in pixels (even number)
[Deafult is:0]=256
 --> 256
Enter starting pixel [Deafult is:33]=
 --> 33
Enter First scan line [Deafult is:1]=
 --> 1
Enter height [Deafult is:320]=256
 --> 256

====>>
width=256,   height=256
StartX=33,   first scan line=1
Want to set a Window?[Y or N] n No

--------- Frame Number = 1 ---------
File will be: H1R?.RV

Include this frame? [Y or N] y Yes
Run Number= 20642
Patient I.D. =1061423
Slice number= 1
Slice (table) index= 0
maximal value= 1005
minimal value= 0

--------- Frame Number = 2 ----------
File will be: H2R?.RV

Include this frame? [Y or N] No
This frame is skipped

--------- Frame Number = 3 ---------
File will be: H3R?.RV

Include this frame? [Y or N]   No
This frame is skipped

--------- Frame Number = 4 ---------
File will be: H4R?.RV

Include this frame? [Y or N]   No
This frame is skipped

--------- Frame Number = 5 ---------
File will be: H5R?.RV

Include this frame? [Y or N]   No
This frame is skipped

--------- Frame Number = 6 ---------
File will be: H6R?.RV

Include this frame? [Y or N] yyy Yes
Run Number= 20642
Patient I.D. =1061423
Slice number= 6
Slice (table) index = -10
maximal value= 1002
minimal value= 0

--------- Frame Number = 7 ---------
File will be: H7R?.RV

Include this frame? [Y or N]   Yes
Run Number= 20642
Patient I.D. =1061423
Slice number= 7
Slice (table) index = -20yyyyyyyyyyyyy
maximal value= 999
minimal value= 0

```
--------- Frame Number = 8 ---------
File will be: H8R?.RV

Include this frame? [ Y or N ]   Yes
Run Number= 20642
Patient I.D. =1061423
Slice number= 8
Slice (table) index = -30
maximal value= 1023
minimal value= 0


--------- Frame Number = 9 ---------
File will be: H9R?.RV

Include this frame? [ Y or N ]   Yes
Run Number= 20642
Patient I.D. =1061423
Slice number= 9
Slice (table) index = -40
maximal value= 1023
minimal value= 0


--------- Frame Number = 10 ---------
File will be: H10R?.RV

Include this frame? [ Y or N ]   Yes
Run Number= 20642
Patient I.D. =1061423
Slice number= 10
Slice (table) index = -50
maximal value= 1023
minimal value= 0


--------- Frame Number = 11 ---------
File will be: H11R?.RV

Include this frame? [ Y or N ]   Yes
Run Number= 20642
Patient I.D. =1061423
Slice number= 11
Slice (table) index = -60
maximal value= 983
minimal value= 0


--------- Frame Number = 12 ---------
File will be: H12R?.RV

Include this frame? [ Y or N ]   Yes
Run Number= 20642
Patient I.D. =1061423
Slice number= 12
Slice (table) index = -70
maximal value= 1023
minimal value= 0
```

```
--------- Frame Number = 13 ---------
File will be: H13R?.RV

Include this frame? [ Y or N ]   Yes
Run Number= 20642
Patient I.D. =1061423
Slice number= 13
Slice (table) index = -80
maximal value= 1023
minimal value= 0


--------- Frame Number = 14 ---------
File will be: H14R?.RV

Include this frame? [ Y or N ]   Yes
Run Number= 20642
Patient I.D. =1061423
Slice number= 14
Slice (table) index = -90
maximal value= 1023
minimal value= 0


--------- Frame Number = 15 ---------
File will be: H15R?.RV

Include this frame? [ Y or N ]   Yes
Run Number= 20642
Patient I.D. =1061423
Slice number= 15
Slice (table) index = -100
maximal value= 1023
minimal value= 0


--------- Frame Number = 16 ---------
File will be: H16R?.RV

Include this frame? [ Y or N ]   Yes
Run Number= 20642
Patient I.D. =1061423
Slice number= 16
Slice (table) index = -110
maximal value= 1023
minimal value= 0


--------- Frame Number = 17 ---------
File will be: H17R?.RV

Include this frame? [ Y or N ]   Yes
Run Number= 20642
Patient I.D. =1061423
Slice number= 17
Slice (table) index = -120
maximal value= 1023
minimal value= 0
```

```
--------- Frame Number = 18 ---------
File will be: H18R?.RV

Include this frame? [ Y or N ]  Yes
Run Number= 20642
Patient I.D. =1061423
Slice number= 18
Slice (table) index = -130
maximal value= 951
minimal value= 0


--------- Frame Number = 19 ---------
File will be: H19R?.RV

Include this frame? [ Y or N ]  Yes
Run Number= 20642
Patient I.D. =1061423
Slice number= 19
Slice (table) index = -140
maximal value= 1023
minimal value= 0


--------- Frame Number = 20 ---------
File will be: H20R?.RV

Include this frame? [ Y or N ]  Yes
Run Number= 20642
Patient I.D. =1061423
Slice number= 20
Slice (table) index = -150
maximal value= 1023
minimal value= 0
```

```
--------- Frame Number = 21 ---------
File will be: H21R?.RV

Include this frame? [ Y or N ]  Yes
Run Number= 20642
Patient I.D. =1061423
Slice number= 21
Slice (table) index = -160
maximal value= 958
minimal value= 0


--------- Frame Number = 22 ---------
File will be: H22R?.RV

Include this frame? [ Y or N ] nnn No
This frame is skipped


--------- Frame Number = 23 ---------
File will be: H23R?.RV

Include this frame? [ Y or N ]  No
This frame is skipped


--------- Frame Number = 24 ---------
File will be: H24R?.RV

Include this frame? [ Y or N ]  No
This frame is skipped


========================================
======= NEW SET OF SLICES =============
========================================

Continue? [ Y or N ] n No
End of SAIL execution
[:04:08   ]
```

D.3 Three-Dimensional Image Structure

In essence, the multiple-resolution 3-D images can be considered a four-dimensional structure, but the different dimensions have distinguished characteristics. The first two dimensions, that correspond to the 2-D individual slices, are "dense," in that all elements are uniformly close to each other. The third dimension, that is referred to here as the *Zlevel,* is sparse and not very uniform. It is called the *inter slice* (or scanning) distance and may change even between slices of the same scan. In addition, because the order of slices does not determine their Z-location, it is termed *index* in the original image. The situation is even more random for the fourth dimension, the resolution. For these reasons it is convenient to arrange the image as a multiple-resolution 3-D image, where each such image is an indexed list of 2-D images, which in our case are RIFF files. The collection of RIFF files is organized as a list of lists of files, and the descriptor of this data structure is stored in a single representative file, called the *image file.* Formally, the structure is defined as follows:

Definition D.1: A 3-d image

$$<image\ file> ::= \{<resolution_1>,...,<resolution_n>\}$$

$$<resolution_i> ::= \{<RIFF_{i,1}>,...,<RIFF_{i,m}>\{$$

$$<RIFF_{i,j}> ::= \text{2-D dense raster image file}$$

where n is the number of resolutions
         m is the number of Zlevels for all resolutions.

The structure in the image file is a dump of a LEAP structure (see Appendix G.1). This LEAP structure is the list of lists of which elements are file names, and which are associated with additional data to describe their geometrical aspects. The RIFF files for a given image are assumed to be in the same file directory as the image file itself. When in main memory, the image actually occupies little space, until *boxes* (or subimages) are read in from the RIFF files (to be described in the next section). The internal image structure consists of the structures in Definition D.1, while the <image> is associated with a header that is accessed via NTV mechanism like headers of RIFF files, for values like the X and Y sizes of each slice (that are demanded to be the same for all slices).

The following is a listed 3-D image structure, which is achieved by traversing the internal list structure. The header of each RIFF file, whose name is encountered in this traversal, is accessed to ensure consistency between the file and its position in the 3-D image. This listing is made for the same image file that was extracted from the scan of Listing D.1.

Listing D.2:

```
=====  3 dimentional image printout
=====

device= ''; PPN= '[,,mtutil]'.
Image contains 3 resolutions:

image Xsize,Ysize= 256, 256


-----    Resolution 1
   resolution factor= 1

Plane  1
     file Name= H21R1.RV.    Zlevel= -160
     in the file:
          Zlevel=-160, Resolution=1
          Xsize= 256, Ysize= 256

Plane  2
     file Name= H20R1.RV.    Zlevel= -150
     in the file:
          Zlevel=-150, Resolution=1
          Xsize= 256, Ysize= 256

Plane  3
     file Name= H19R1.RV.    Zlevel= -140
     in the file:
          Zlevel=-140, Resolution=1
          Xsize= 256, Ysize= 256

Plane  4
     file Name= H18R1.RV.    Zlevel= -130
     in the file:
          Zlevel=-130, Resolution=1
          Xsize= 256, Ysize= 256

Plane  5
     file Name= H17R1.RV.    Zlevel= -120
     in the file:
          Zlevel=-120, Resolution=1
          Xsize= 256, Ysize= 256

Plane  6
     file Name= H16R1.RV.    Zlevel= -110
     in the file:
          Zlevel=-110, Resolution=1
          Xsize= 256, Ysize= 256

Plane  7
     file Name= H15R1.RV.    Zlevel= -100
     in the file:
          Zlevel=-100, Resolution=1
          Xsize= 256, Ysize= 256

Plane  8
     file Name= H14R1.RV.    Zlevel= -90
     in the file:
          Zlevel=-90, Resolution=1
          Xsize= 256, Ysize= 256

Plane  9
     file Name= H13R1.RV.    Zlevel= -80
     in the file:
          Zlevel=-80, Resolution=1
          Xsize= 256, Ysize= 256

Plane  10
     file Name= H12R1.RV.    Zlevel= -70
     in the file:
          Zlevel=-70, Resolution=1
          Xsize= 256, Ysize= 256

Plane  11
     file Name= H11R1.RV.    Zlevel= -60
     in the file:
          Zlevel=-60, Resolution=1
          Xsize= 256, Ysize= 256

Plane  12
     file Name= H10R1.RV.    Zlevel= -50
     in the file:
          Zlevel=-50, Resolution=1
          Xsize= 256, Ysize= 256

Plane  13
     file Name= H9R1.RV.    Zlevel= -40
     in the file:
          Zlevel=-40, Resolution=1
          Xsize= 256, Ysize= 256

Plane  14
     file Name= H8R1.RV.    Zlevel= -30
     in the file:
          Zlevel=-30, Resolution=1
          Xsize= 256, Ysize= 256

Plane  15
     file Name= H7R1.RV.    Zlevel= -20
     in the file:
          Zlevel=-20, Resolution=1
          Xsize= 256, Ysize= 256

Plane  16
     file Name= H6R1.RV.    Zlevel= -10
     in the file:
          Zlevel=-10, Resolution=1
          Xsize= 256, Ysize= 256

Plane  17
     file Name= H1R1.RV.    Zlevel= 0
     in the file:
          Zlevel=0, Resolution=1
          Xsize= 256, Ysize= 256


-----    Resolution 2
   resolution factor= 4

Plane  1
     file Name= H21R2.RV.    Zlevel= -160
     in the file:
          Zlevel=-160, Resolution=4
          Xsize= 256, Ysize= 256

Plane  2
     file Name= H20R2.RV.    Zlevel= -150
     in the file:
          Zlevel=-150, Resolution=4
          Xsize= 256, Ysize= 256
```

```
Plane  3
     file Name= H19R2.RV.    Zlevel= -140
     in the file:
          Zlevel=-140, Resolution=4
          Xsize= 256, Ysize= 256

Plane  4
     file Name= H18R2.RV.    Zlevel= -130
     in the file:
          Zlevel=-130, Resolution=4
          Xsize= 256, Ysize= 256

Plane  5
     file Name= H17R2.RV.    Zlevel= -120
     in the file:
          Zlevel=-120, Resolution=4
          Xsize= 256, Ysize= 256

Plane  6
     file Name= H16R2.RV.    Zlevel= -110
     in the file:
          Zlevel=-110, Resolution=4
          Xsize= 256, Ysize= 256

Plane  7
     file Name= H15R2.RV.    Zlevel= -100
     in the file:
          Zlevel=-100, Resolution=4
          Xsize= 256, Ysize= 256

Plane  8
     file Name= H14R2.RV.    Zlevel= -90
     in the file:
          Zlevel=-90, Resolution=4
          Xsize= 256, Ysize= 256

Plane  9
     file Name= H13R2.RV.    Zlevel= -80
     in the file:
          Zlevel=-80, Resolution=4
          Xsize= 256, Ysize= 256

Plane  10
     file Name= H12R2.RV.    Zlevel= -70
     in the file:
          Zlevel=-70, Resolution=4
          Xsize= 256, Ysize= 256

Plane  11
     file Name= H11R2.RV.    Zlevel= -60
     in the file:
          Zlevel=-60, Resolution=4
          Xsize= 256, Ysize= 256

Plane  12
     file Name= H10R2.RV.    Zlevel= -50
     in the file:
          Zlevel=-50, Resolution=4
          Xsize= 256, Ysize= 256

Plane  13
     file Name= H9R2.RV.    Zlevel= -40
     in the file:
          Zlevel=-40, Resolution=4
          Xsize= 256, Ysize= 256
```

```
Plane  14
     file Name= H8R2.RV.    Zlevel= -30
     in the file:
          Zlevel=-30, Resolution=4
          Xsize= 256, Ysize= 256

Plane  15
     file Name= H7R2.RV.    Zlevel= -20
     in the file:
          Zlevel=-20, Resolution=4
          Xsize= 256, Ysize= 256

Plane  16
     file Name= H6R2.RV.    Zlevel= -10
     in the file:
          Zlevel=-10, Resolution=4
          Xsize= 256, Ysize= 256

Plane  17
     file Name= H1R2.RV.    Zlevel= 0
     in the file:
          Zlevel=0, Resolution=4
          Xsize= 256, Ysize= 256


-----    Resolution  3
     resolution factor= 16

Plane  1
     file Name= H21R3.RV.    Zlevel= -160
     in the file:
          Zlevel=-160, Resolution=16
          Xsize= 256, Ysize= 256

Plane  2
     file Name= H20R3.RV.    Zlevel= -150
     in the file:
          Zlevel=-150, Resolution=16
          Xsize= 256, Ysize= 256

Plane  3
     file Name= H19R3.RV.    Zlevel= -140
     in the file:
     Zlevel=-140, Resolution=16
          Xsize= 256, Ysize= 256

Plane  4
     file Name= H18R3.RV.    Zlevel= -130
     in the file:
          Zlevel=-130, Resolution=16
          Xsize= 256, Ysize= 256

Plane  5
     file Name= H17R3.RV.    Zlevel= -120
     in the file:
          Zlevel=-120, Resolution=16
          Xsize= 256, Ysize= 256

Plane  6
     file Name= H16R3.RV.    Zlevel= -110
     in the file:
          Zlevel=-110, Resolution=16
          Xsize= 256, Ysize= 256
```

Plane 7
     file Name= H15R3.RV.   Zlevel= -100
     in the file:
          Zlevel=-100, Resolution=16
          Xsize= 256, Ysize= 256

Plane 8
     file Name= H14R3.RV.   Zlevel= -90
     in the file:
          Zlevel=-90, Resolution=16
          Xsize= 256, Ysize= 256

Plane 9
     file Name= H13R3.RV.   Zlevel= -80
     in the file:
          Zlevel=-80, Resolution=16
          Xsize= 256, Ysize= 256

Plane 10
     file Name= H12R3.RV.   Zlevel= -70
     in the file:
          Zlevel=-70, Resolution=16
          Xsize= 256, Ysize= 256

Plane 11
     file Name= H11R3.RV.   Zlevel= -60
     in the file:
          Zlevel=-60, Resolution=16
          Xsize= 256, Ysize= 256

Plane 12
     file Name= H10R3.RV.   Zlevel= -50
     in the file:
          Zlevel=-50, Resolution=16
          Xsize= 256, Ysize= 256

Plane 13
     file Name= H9R3.RV.   Zlevel= -40
     in the file:
          Zlevel=-40, Resolution=16
          Xsize= 256, Ysize= 256

Plane 14
     file Name= H8R3.RV.   Zlevel= -30
     in the file:
          Zlevel=-30, Resolution=16
          Xsize= 256, Ysize= 256

Plane 15
     file Name= H7R3.RV.   Zlevel= -20
     in the file:
          Zlevel=-20, Resolution=16
          Xsize= 256, Ysize= 256

Plane 16
     file Name= H6R3.RV.   Zlevel= -10
     in the file:
          Zlevel=-10, Resolution=16
          Xsize= 256, Ysize= 256

Plane 17
     file Name= H1R3.RV.   Zlevel= 0
     in the file:
          Zlevel=0, Resolution=16
          Xsize= 256, Ysize= 256
End of SAIL execution
[14.23   ]

D.4 Image Access

To access the image, a box must be created in the main memory—a box of some limited size, out of the total image, and in some resolution. Once a box is created, image values are accessible as the function of real coordinates $[x,y,z]$. A voxel occupies for different resolutions a different-sized volume, or a "territory." The relation between corresponding voxels of different resolutions implies some rules for defining these territories. To demonstrate that calculation, a 2-D analogy is depicted in Figure D.4.

Each pixel is addressed via some index (i,j). For example, the (0,0) pixel of resolution-factor 4 is the average of pixels (0,0),(0,1),(1,0),(1,1) of resolution-factor 1. But, while the area related to pixel (0,0) in resolution-factor 1 is the rectangle (defined by coordinates of two opposite corners)

$$\left(-\frac{1}{2},\ -\frac{1}{2}\right) - \left(\frac{1}{2},\ \frac{1}{2}\right),$$

the area covered by the (0,0) pixel of resolution-factor 4 is

$$\left(-\frac{1}{2},\ -\frac{1}{2}\right) - \left(1\frac{1}{2},\ 1\frac{1}{2}\right).$$

For a given resolution, a real numbered coordinate (x,y) is in pixel (i,j), if it falls into the area covered by it (its territory), and the formula per coordinate is

$$i = Floor\left[\frac{x + \frac{1}{2}}{<resolution\ factor>}\right]. \tag{D.1}$$

A similar formula will do for j (via y). The inverse conversion and additional useful formulae are:

1. Converting an index of a pixel to the real coordinate of its center (the pixel territory size is half the resolution factor on both sides of its center),

$$x = <resolution\ factor> \cdot \left[i + \frac{1}{2}\right] - \frac{1}{2} \tag{D.2}$$

2. Converting a real coordinate x to the index of the pixel "above" it,

$$C_i = 1 + Floor \left[\frac{x + \frac{1}{2}}{< resolution\ factor > - \frac{1}{2}} \right] \qquad (D.3)$$

3. Converting a real coordinate x to the index of the pixel "below" it,

$$F_i = Floor \left[\frac{x + \frac{1}{2}}{< reslution\ factor > - \frac{1}{2}} \right]. \qquad (D.4)$$

A box (3-D subimage) consists of a list of arrays, and it is associated with a descriptor that contains the box dimensions in X, Y, and Z, and the Zlevels for each of the 2-D image arrays in the list. An image value can be randomly accessed in two ways, either directly or by interpolation. The direct-access technique is to return the value of the pixel whose territory contains the given coordinate; the interpolation scheme is depicted in Figure D.4. The four (eight in the case of 3-D) pixels (voxels in 3-D) on both sides of the given coordinate in all directions (via Formulae D.3 and D.4) are averaged, weighted by the inverse of the distance of their centers from the given coordinate. For the example in Figure D.4, the interpolated value at location (x_1, y_1) (refer to Figure D.1) is as follows:

$$Value\,(x_1, y_1) = \left(x_1 - \frac{1}{2} \right) \cdot Average_y\,(y_1, 1) + \left(2\frac{1}{2} - x_1 \right) \cdot Average_y\,(y_1, 0) \qquad (D.5)$$

where

$$Average_y\,(y_1, i) = \left(y_1 - \frac{1}{2} \right) \cdot P_{i,1} + \left(2\frac{1}{2} - y_1 \right) \cdot P_{i,0}$$

and $P_{i,j}$ is pixel value of index (i,j).

Of course, the numbers $\frac{1}{2}$ and $2\frac{1}{2}$ in that example are based in the location of $[x_1, y_1]$ and are generally obtained via Formulae D.3 and D.4.

Given that mechanism for the random access of image values in a box, any planar cross section of the image is attainable and can be displayed. To demonstrate the effect of the various resolution images under the two access methods, Figure D.5 presents a stack of slices in an artistic fashion for resolution factors 4 and 16, for these two access methods.

Figure D.5.   3-D images of resolutions 4 and 16, for both interpolation and noninterpolation access of image values, for arbitrary real coordinates. A) Resolution factor 4 without interpolation; and B) Resolution factor 4 with interpolation; (continued on next page).

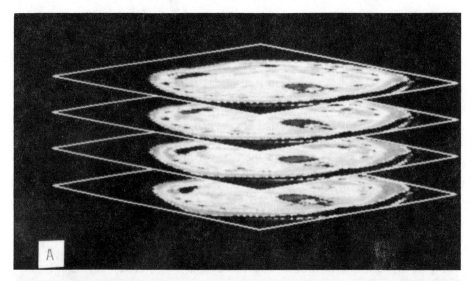

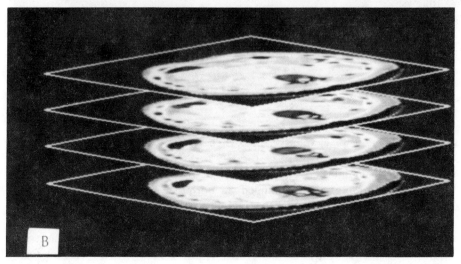

Figure D.5. (continued): C) Resolution factor 16 without interpolation; and D) Resolution factor 16 with interpolation.

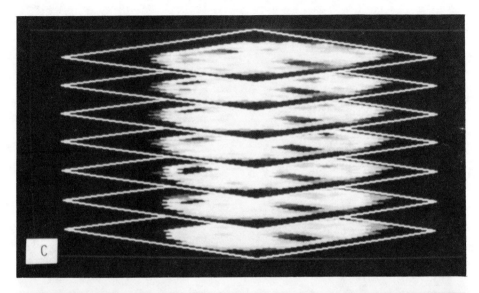

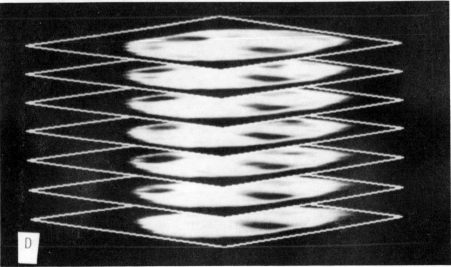

Figure D.6 represents most of the slices of the other two sets of CAT images (out of the three set of slices used in this thesis, of which the first set is presented in Figure 1.3).

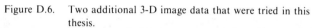

Figure D.6.   Two additional 3-D image data that were tried in this
thesis.

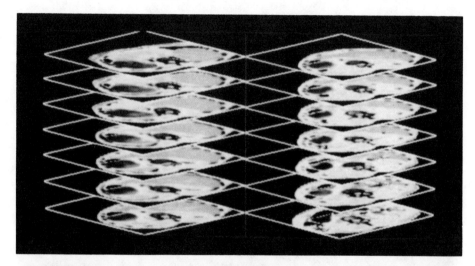

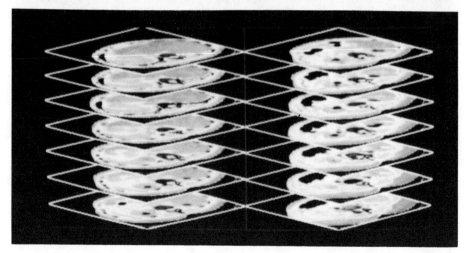

Appendix E

Results Tracing

E.1 Introduction

The program is capable of tracing the fitting process and printing the effect of activating experts in the various model levels, the returned results, and the amount of resources spent for each of them. The trace-listing is indented whenever a new model level is entered, and all elements of the same level are enumerated. The expert name of the corresponding level is printed, together with all the nonzero resources spent. The counted resources are Disk I/O for Reads (RD) and Writes (WR), the CPU time (CPU), and elapsed real time (RTIME). The time resources needed are greater when the program is running with debug facilities ON; they are even greater when the graphics option is selected. After the model is traversed in search and result-propagation cycles, the performed modifications are printed before the next iteration starts. On exiting an expert, the returned results are printed and annotated via the following legend:

Conf	— Total confidence;
Dcnf	— Displacement (translation) confidence;
Scnf	— Scale confidence;
Dx	— Displacement (translation) in the X direction;
Dy	— Displacement (translation) in the Y direction;
Dz	— Displacement (translation) in the Z direction;
Sx	— Scale in the X direction;
Sy	— Scale in the Y direction;
Sz	— Scale in the Z direction; and
Orientation	— Orientation vector (in 3-D).

All these result types are returned by organ experts, while lower level experts return only a corresponding subset.

The pyramid-of-resolution principle is reflected in the trace by preceding every fitting effort for an image of a given resolution by the line

*** RESOLUTION is: n ***

where n is 16, 4, and 1. A fitting problem at a given resolution is terminated when the organ-level criteria are met, and also the cross-section-level criteria are either met or are not allowed when the resolution is too coarse. When a fitting problem is completed, the line "No more changes at all !!" is printed in the trace.

The following trace was recorded in locating the left kidney of the first 3-D image, which is also presented in Figure 7.3. The trace is composed of three parts. Listing E.1 is a full trace (down to the boundary-point level) of the search in a single cross section. It is intended to demonstrate the amount of resources used there. Listing E.2 is a full trace of a fitting process, where traces are limited to the cross sections only, for which the resource report is inhibited to keep the listing size down. The third is Listing E.3, which represents only the modifications and their values in the various levels as they occurred during the search.

In this trace, model nodes are named as follows:

—The organ node is "Left Kidney,"

—Cross-section nodes are "LKDNYi," where i= 1,2, ...,9, and

—Boundary-point nodes are named after the corresponding activated expert, like "Back Gradient," and so forth.

All modifications are announced in terms which are relative to the geometric situation when they occur. In Listing E.2, they are usually followed with a statement of the appropriate new geometric situation. In general (as for Listing E.3) the new geometric situation for size, location, and orientation can be calculated by concatenating all relative modifications.

Timing: Notable is the CPU time utilization. A complete organ fit takes about 8 minutes CPU and about 40 minutes of elapsed time. A single boundary search takes a small fraction of a CPU second, while a complete cross-section search takes 1 to 2 CPU seconds. This suggests that in a truly parallel environment the parallel processing option (see 4.2.1) could conceivably reduce the time for a cross-section scan to a small fraction of a second, collapsing the search time for a full kidney scan from a third of a minute to less then a second, and reducing the total fitting time for a search of the kidney to a few seconds of parallel CPU time.

Listing E.1: Cross-section trace:

```
5).  ENTERING LKDNY5
  1).  ENTERING Gradient
  1).  EXITING Gradient.
       Resources: WR= 0, RD= 0,
                  CPU= 0.34, RTIME= 0.33,
       Results are: Conf= 1.000, Dx= -5.000,

  2).  ENTERING Gradient
  2).  EXITING Gradient.
       Resources: WR= 1, RD= 0,
                  CPU= 0.22, RTIME= 0.33,
       Results are: Conf= 1.000, Dx= -1.000,

  3).  ENTERING Gradient
  3).  EXITING Gradient.
       Resources: WR= 0, RD= 0,
                  CPU= 0.17, RTIME= 0.17,
       Results are: Conf= 1.000, Dx= 1.000,

  4).  ENTERING Gradient
  4).  EXITING Gradient.
       Resources: WR= 0, RD= 0,
                  CPU= 0.17, RTIME= 0.17,
       Results are: Conf= 1.000, Dx= 2.000,

  5).  ENTERING Gradient
  5).  EXITING Gradient.
       Resources: WR= 0, RD= 0,
                  CPU= 0.17, RTIME= 0.16,
       Results are: Conf= 1.000, Dx= 5.000,

  6).  ENTERING Gradient
  6).  EXITING Gradient.
       Resources: WR= 0, RD= 0,
                  CPU= 0.17, RTIME= 0.16,
       Results are: Conf= 1.000, Dx= 8.000,

  7).  ENTERING DontCare
  7).  EXITING DontCare.
       Resources: WR= 0, RD= 0,
                  CPU= 0.0, RTIME= 0.0,
       Results are: Conf= .000, Dx= .000,

  8).  ENTERING DontCare
  8).  EXITING DontCare.
       Resources: WR= 0, RD= 0,
                  CPU= 0.0, RTIME= 0.0,
       Results are: Conf= .000, Dx= .000,

  9).  ENTERING DontCare
  9).  EXITING DontCare.
       Resources: WR= 0, RD= 0,
                  CPU= 0.14, RTIME= 0.16,
       Results are: Conf= .000, Dx= .000,

 10).  ENTERING DontCare
 10).  EXITING DontCare.
       Resources: WR= 0, RD= 0,
                  CPU= 0.0, RTIME= 0.0,
       Results are: Conf= .000, Dx= .000,

 11).  ENTERING DontCare
 11).  EXITING DontCare.
       Resources: WR= 0, RD= 0,
                  CPU= 0.0, RTIME= 0.0,
       Results are: Conf= .000, Dx= .000,

 12).  ENTERING Back Gradient
 12).  EXITING Back Gradient.
       Resources: WR= 0, RD= 0,
                  CPU= 0.36, RTIME= 0.34,
       Results are: Conf= 1.000, Dx= -7.000,

 13).  ENTERING Back Gradient
 13).  EXITING Back Gradient.
       Resources: WR= 1, RD= 0,
                  CPU= 0.17, RTIME= 0.17,
       Results are: Conf= 1.000, Dx= -10.000,

 14).  ENTERING Back Gradient
 14).  EXITING Back Gradient.
       Resources: WR= 0, RD= 0,
                  CPU= 0.17, RTIME= 0.17,
       Results are: Conf= 1.000, Dx= -13.000,

 15).  ENTERING Back Gradient
 15).  EXITING Back Gradient.
       Resources: WR= 0, RD= 0,
                  CPU= 0.17, RTIME= 0.17,
       Results are: Conf= 1.000, Dx= -12.000,

 16).  ENTERING Back Gradient
 16).  EXITING Back Gradient.
       Resources: WR= 1, RD= 0,
                  CPU= 0.32, RTIME= 0.50,
       Results are: Conf= 1.000, Dx= -13.000,

 17).  ENTERING Back Gradient
 17).  EXITING Back Gradient.
       Resources: WR= 0, RD= 0,
                  CPU= 0.17, RTIME= 0.16,
       Results are: Conf= 1.000, Dx= -13.000,

 18).  ENTERING Back Gradient
 18).  EXITING Back Gradient.
       Resources: WR= 0, RD= 0,
                  CPU= 0.33, RTIME= 0.34,
       Results are: Conf= 1.000, Dx= -12.000,

 19).  ENTERING Back Gradient
 19).  EXITING Back Gradient.
       Resources: WR= 0, RD= 0,
                  CPU= 0.29, RTIME= 0.34,
       Results are: Conf= 1.000, Dx= -11.000,

 20).  ENTERING Back Gradient
 20).  EXITING Back Gradient.
       Resources: WR= 0, RD= 0,
                  CPU= 0.36, RTIME= 0.33,
       Results are: Conf= 1.000, Dx= -10.000,

 21).  ENTERING Back Gradient
 21).  EXITING Back Gradient.
       Resources: WR= 1, RD= 0,
                  CPU= 0.41, RTIME= 0.66,
       Results are: Conf= 1.000, Dx= -8.000,

 22).  ENTERING Back Gradient
 22).  EXITING Back Gradient.
       Resources: WR= 0,
                  CPU= 0.17,        0.17,
       Results are: Conf= 1.0         -5.000,

  5).  EXITING LKDNY5.
       Resources: WR= 8, RD= 0,
                  CPU= 1.554, RTIME= 1.783,
       Results are: Conf= .773,
       Dx= -.439, Dy= 5.622, Dz= .000,
       Dist= -7.500, Scale= .643,
```

Listing E.2: Full left-kidney trace

```
 1). ENTERING Main Block
***   RESOLUTION IS: 16   ***

 1). ENTERING Left Kidney
 1). EXITING Left Kidney.
       Resources: WR= 1, RD= 16,
                  CPU= 0.555, RTIME= 22.233,
       Results are: Conf= .000, Dcnf= .000, Dx= .000,
       Dz= .000, Dy= .000, Scnf= .000,
       Sx= 1.000, Sy= 1.000, Sz= 1.000,
       Orientation = [.000, .000, 1.000]

Organ - No changes

No more changes at all !!

***   RESOLUTION IS: 4   ***

 2). ENTERING Left Kidney
 1). EXITING LKDNY1. Results are: Conf= .714,
       Dx= 4.037, Dy= 1.958, Dz= .000,
       Dist= -5.000, Scale= .167,
 2). EXITING LKDNY2. Results are: Conf= .909,
       Dx= .942, Dy= 3.478, Dz= .000,
       Dist= -2.727, Scale= .727,
 3). EXITING LKDNY3. Results are: Conf= 1.000,
       Dx= 1.663, Dy= 5.368, Dz= .000,
       Dist= -2.889, Scale= .819,
 4). EXITING LKDNY4. Results are: Conf= .810,
       Dx= 1.340, Dy= 5.038, Dz= .000,
       Dist= -6.385, Scale= .681,
 5). EXITING LKDNY5. Results are: Conf= .773,
       Dx= -.875, Dy= 6.085, Dz= .000,
       Dist= -7.077, Scale= .663,
 6). EXITING LKDNY6. Results are: Conf= .810,
       Dx= .658, Dy= 4.792, Dz= .000,
       Dist= -5.375, Scale= .731,
 7). EXITING LKDNY7. Results are: Conf= 1.000,
       Dx= 2.871, Dy= 3.621, Dz= .000,
       Dist= -.938, Scale= .941,
 8). EXITING LKDNY8. Results are: Conf= .909,
       Dx= .734, Dy= 1.018, Dz= .000,
       Dist= -1.519, Scale= .848,
 9). EXITING LKDNY9. Results are: Conf= 1.000,
       Dx= -.457, Dy= -.602, Dz= .000,
       Dist= 2.500, Scale= 1.417,

10). EXITING Zscan of LKDNY1.
       Results are: Conf= .714, Zdisp= 1.000,
11). EXITING Zscan of LKDNY9.
       Results are: Conf= .571, Zdisp= .000,

 2). EXITING Left Kidney.
       Resources: WR= 1, RD= 53,
                  CPU= 16.35, RTIME= 48.50,
       Results are: Conf= .722, Dcnf= .722, Dx= 1.172,
       Dz= .000, Dy= 5.088, Scnf= .000,
       Sx= 1.000, Sy= 1.000, Sz= 1.000,
       Orientation = [-.016, -.011, 1.000, ]

Org disp( 1.1723223, 5.0880070, .0000000),
 new center is: (81.1723220, 75.0880070,-70.0000000).

 3). ENTERING Left Kidney
 1). EXITING LKDNY1. Results are: Conf= .714,
       Dx= -.377, Dy= .911, Dz= .000,
       Dist= .810, Scale= 1.135,
```

```
 2). EXITING LKDNY2. Results are: Conf= 1.000,
       Dx= .177, Dy= .871, Dz= .000,
       Dist= -.308, Scale= .969,
 3). EXITING LKDNY3. Results are: Conf= 1.000,
       Dx= 1.295, Dy= 1.104, Dz= .000,
       Dist= -2.450, Scale= .847,
 4). EXITING LKDNY4. Results are: Conf= .810,
       Dx= -.072, Dy= 1.038, Dz= .000,
       Dist= -2.929, Scale= .854,
 5). EXITING LKDNY5. Results are: Conf= .773,
       Dx= -.241, Dy= 2.428, Dz= .000,
       Dist= -4.000, Scale= .810,
 6). EXITING LKDNY6. Results are: Conf= .810,
       Dx= .483, Dy= 3.323, Dz= .000,
       Dist= -3.529, Scale= .824,
 7). EXITING LKDNY7. Results are: Conf= 1.000,
       Dx= 1.535, Dy= 1.462, Dz= .000,
       Dist= -.889, Scale= .944,
 8). EXITING LKDNY8. Results are: Conf= .909,
       Dx= -.292, Dy= -.367, Dz= .000,
       Dist= .900, Scale= 1.090,
 9). EXITING LKDNY9. Results are: Conf= 1.000,
       Dx= -1.704, Dy= -.444, Dz= .000,
       Dist= 3.200, Scale= 1.533,

10). EXITING Zscan of LKDNY1.
       Results are: Conf= 1.000, Zdisp= 1.000,
11). EXITING Zscan of LKDNY9.
       Results are: Conf= .714, Zdisp= 10.000,

 3). EXITING Left Kidney.
       Resources: WR= 0, RD= 199,
                  CPU= 17.530, RTIME= 48.516,
       Results are: Conf= .857, Dcnf= .857, Dx= .000,
       Dz= 5.000, Dy= .000, Scnf= .000,
       Sx= 1.000, Sy= 1.000, Sz= 1.000,
       Orientation= -[.006, .006, 1.000]

Org disp( .0000000, .0000000, 5.0000000),
 new center is: (81.1723220, 75.0880070,-65.0000000).

 4). ENTERING Left Kidney
 1). EXITING LKDNY1. Results are: Conf= .857,
       Dx= -2.474, Dy= -.116, Dz= .000,
       Dist= 3.500, Scale= 1.583,
 2). EXITING LKDNY2. Results are: Conf= 1.000,
       Dx= .177, Dy= .871, Dz= .000,
       Dist= -.308, Scale= .969,
 3). EXITING LKDNY3. Results are: Conf= 1.000,
       Dx= 1.295, Dy= 1.104, Dz= .000,
       Dist= -2.450, Scale= .847,
 4). EXITING LKDNY4. Results are: Conf= .810,
       Dx= -.072, Dy= 1.038, Dz= .000,
       Dist= -2.929, Scale= .854,
 5). EXITING LKDNY5. Results are: Conf= .773,
       Dx= -.241, Dy= 2.428, Dz= .000,
       Dist= -4.000, Scale= .810,
 6). EXITING LKDNY6. Results are: Conf= .810,
       Dx= .483, Dy= 3.323, Dz= .000,
       Dist= -3.529, Scale= .824,
 7). EXITING LKDNY7. Results are: Conf= 1.000,
       Dx= 1.535, Dy= 1.462, Dz= .000,
       Dist= -.889, Scale= .944,
 8). EXITING LKDNY8. Results are: Conf= .909,
       Dx= -.292, Dy= -.367, Dz= .000,
       Dist= .900, Scale= 1.090,
```

9). EXITING LKDNY9. Results are: Conf= 1.000,
     Dx= .255, Dy= -.700, Dz= .000,
     Dist= 3.000, Scale= 1.500,

10). EXITING Zscan of LKDNY1.
     Results are: Conf= 1.000, Zdisp= -4.000,
11). EXITING Zscan of LKDNY9.
     Results are: Conf= .714, Zdisp= 5.000,

4). EXITING Left Kidney.
     Resources: WR= 0, RD= 164,
          CPU= 17.333, RTIME= 59.516,
     Results are: Conf= .857, Dcnf= .000, Dx= .000,
     Dz= .000, Dy= .000, Scnf= .857,
     Sx= 1.000, Sy= 1.000, Sz= 1.100,
     Orientation= [.017, .010, 1.000]

Org scale (1.0000000, 1.0000000, 1.1000000)
  new size: (40.000000 40.000000 88.000000).

5). ENTERING Left Kidney

1). EXITING LKDNY1. Results are: Conf= .857,
     Dx= -2.474, Dy= -.116, Dz= .000,
     Dist= 3.500, Scale= 1.583,
2). EXITING LKDNY2. Results are: Conf= 1.000,
     Dx= .177, Dy= .871, Dz= .000,
     Dist= -.308, Scale= .969,
3). EXITING LKDNY3. Results are: Conf= 1.000,
     Dx= 1.295, Dy= 1.104, Dz= .000,
     Dist= -2.450, Scale= .847,
4). EXITING LKDNY4. Results are: Conf= .810,
     Dx= -.072, Dy= 1.038, Dz= .000,
     Dist= -2.929, Scale= .854,
5). EXITING LKDNY5. Results are: Conf= .773,
     Dx= -.241, Dy= 2.428, Dz= .000,
     Dist= -4.000, Scale= .810,
6). EXITING LKDNY6. Results are: Conf= .810,
     Dx= 2.233, Dy= 3.059, Dz= .000,
     Dist= -5.556, Scale= .722,
7). EXITING LKDNY7. Results are: Conf= 1.000,
     Dx= 3.330, Dy= 2.242, Dz= .000,
     Dist= -3.000, Scale= .813,
8). EXITING LKDNY8. Results are: Conf= 1.000,
     Dx= 1.662, Dy= .612, Dz= .000,
     Dist= -1.719, Scale= .828,
9). EXITING LKDNY9. Results are: Conf= 1.000,
     Dx= .255, Dy= -.700, Dz= .000,
     Dist= 3.000, Scale= 1.500,

10). EXITING Zscan of LKDNY1.
     Results are: Conf= 1.000, Zdisp= -1.000,
11). EXITING Zscan of LKDNY9.
     Results are: Conf= .714, Zdisp= 1.000,

5). EXITING Left Kidney.
     Resources: WR= 0, RD= 121,
          CPU= 16.797, RTIME= 39.483,
     Results are: Conf= .667, Dcnf= .000, Dx= .000,
     Dz= .000, Dy= .000, Scnf= .667,
     Sx= .900, Sy= .900, Sz= 1.000,
     Orientation= [.043, .017, .999]

Organ - No changes

No more changes at all !!

*** RESOLUTION IS: 1 ***

6). ENTERING Left Kidney
1). EXITING LKDNY1. Results are: Conf= 1.000,
     Dx= -2.049, Dy= -.807, Dz= .000,
     Dist= 4.400, Scale= 1.733,
2). EXITING LKDNY2. Results are: Conf= 1.000,
     Dx= -.349, Dy= .864, Dz= .000,
     Dist= .364, Scale= 1.036,
3). EXITING LKDNY3. Results are: Conf= 1.000,
     Dx= .596, Dy= 1.177, Dz= .000,
     Dist= -2.526, Scale= .842,
4). EXITING LKDNY4. Results are: Conf= .810,
     Dx= .069, Dy= 2.610, Dz= .000,
     Dist= -3.571, Scale= .821,
5). EXITING LKDNY5. Results are: Conf= .773,
     Dx= .147, Dy= 2.728, Dz= .000,
     Dist= -3.444, Scale= .836,
6). EXITING LKDNY6. Results are: Conf= .810,
     Dx= .595, Dy= 2.657, Dz= .000,
     Dist= -4.444, Scale= .778,
7). EXITING LKDNY7. Results are: Conf= 1.000,
     Dx= 1.645, Dy= .625, Dz= .000,
     Dist= -3.533, Scale= .779,
8). EXITING LKDNY8. Results are: Conf= 1.000,
     Dx= 1.347, Dy= 1.018, Dz= .000,
     Dist= -2.276, Scale= .772,
9). EXITING LKDNY9. Results are: Conf= 1.000,
     Dx= .000, Dy= -.373, Dz= .000,
     Dist= .462, Scale= 1.077,

10). EXITING Zscan of LKDNY1.
     Results are: Conf= .857, Zdisp= -1.000,

11). EXITING Zscan of LKDNY9.
     Results are: Conf= .571, Zdisp= 1.000,

6). EXITING Left Kidney.
     Resources: WR= 0, RD= 423,
          CPU= 17.664, RTIME= 1:3.516,
     Results are: Conf= .833, Dcnf= .611, Dx= .368,
     Dz= .000, Dy= 1.177, Scnf= .833,
     Sx= .900, Sy= .900, Sz= 1.025,
     Orientation= [.027, .014, 1.000]
Org disp(1.0000000, 1.1769352, .0000000),
  new center is: (82.1723220, 76.2649420,-65.0000000).

7). ENTERING Left Kidney
1). EXITING LKDNY1. Results are: Conf= 1.000,
     Dx= -.722, Dy= -.821, Dz= .000,
     Dist= 4.889, Scale= 1.815,
2). EXITING LKDNY2. Results are: Conf= 1.000,
     Dx= -.822, Dy= .447, Dz= .000,
     Dist= 1.636, Scale= 1.164,
3). EXITING LKDNY3. Results are: Conf= 1.000,
     Dx= .045, Dy= .493, Dz= .000,
     Dist= -.778, Scale= .951,
4). EXITING LKDNY4. Results are: Conf= .810,
     Dx= -.262, Dy= 1.510, Dz= .000,
     Dist= -1.875, Scale= .906,
5). EXITING LKDNY5. Results are: Conf= .773,
     Dx= -.215, Dy= 2.232, Dz= .000,
     Dist= -3.000, Scale= .857,
6). EXITING LKDNY6. Results are: Conf= .810,
     Dx= -.046, Dy= 2.083, Dz= .000,
     Dist= -3.235, Scale= .838,
7). EXITING LKDNY7. Results are: Conf= 1.000,
     Dx= 1.483, Dy= .919, Dz= .000,
     Dist= -3.000, Scale= .813,
8). EXITING LKDNY8. Results are: Conf= 1.000,
     Dx= .527, Dy= -.285, Dz= .000,
     Dist= -1.381, Scale= .862,

9). EXITING LKDNY9. Results are: Conf= 1.000,
    Dx= -.520, Dy= -.800, Dz= .000,
    Dist= 2.250, Scale= 1.375,

10). EXITING Zscan of LKDNY1.
    Results are: Conf= 1.000, Zdisp= -1.000,
11). EXITING Zscan of LKDNY9.
    Results are: Conf= .857, Zdisp= 1.000,

7). EXITING Left Kidney.
    Resources: WR= 0, RD= 0,
              CPU= 15.597, RTIME= 39.917,
    Results are: Conf= .929, Dcnf= .667, Dx= -.109,
    Dz= .000, Dy= 1.183, Scnf= .929,
    Sx= .955, Sy= .955, Sz= 1.025,
    Orientation= [.015, .009, 1.000]

Org disp(-1.0000000, 1.1833906, .0000000),
    new center is: (81.1723220, 77.4483330,-65.0000000).

8). ENTERING Left Kidney
    1). EXITING LKDNY1. Results are: Conf= 1.000,
        Dx= -1.060, Dy= .436, Dz= .000,
        Dist= 5.000, Scale= 1.833,
    2). EXITING LKDNY2. Results are: Conf= 1.000,
        Dx= .113, Dy= .077, Dz= .000,
        Dist= 1.500, Scale= 1.150,
    3). EXITING LKDNY3. Results are: Conf= 1.000,
        Dx= -.031, Dy= 1.360, Dz= .000,
        Dist= -.471, Scale= .971,
    4). EXITING LKDNY4. Results are: Conf= .810,
        Dx= .348, Dy= .821, Dz= .000,
        Dist= -2.625, Scale= .869,
    5). EXITING LKDNY5. Results are: Conf= .773,
        Dx= -.183, Dy= 1.989, Dz= .000,
        Dist= -1.476, Scale= .930,
    6). EXITING LKDNY6. Results are: Conf= .810,
        Dx= 1.718, Dy= 1.295, Dz= .000,
        Dist= -3.682, Scale= .816,
    7). EXITING LKDNY7. Results are: Conf= 1.000,
        Dx= .311, Dy= .611, Dz= .000,
        Dist= -2.438, Scale= .848,
    8). EXITING LKDNY8. Results are: Conf= 1.000,
        Dx= 1.882, Dy= -.563, Dz= .000,
        Dist= .000, Scale= 1.000,
    9). EXITING LKDNY9. Results are: Conf= .857,
        Dx= 1.867, Dy= -1.178, Dz= .000,
        Dist= -2.158, Scale= .640,

    10). EXITING Zscan of LKDNY1.
        Results are: Conf= 1.000, Zdisp= -1.000,
    11). EXITING Zscan of LKDNY9.
        Results are: Conf= .571, Zdisp= 1.000,

8). EXITING Left Kidney.
    Resources: WR= 0, RD= 0,
              CPU= 14.231, RTIME= 39.400,
    Results are: Conf= .786, Dcnf= .778, Dx= .177,
    Dz= .000, Dy= 1.018, Scnf= .786,
    Sx= .957, Sy= .957, Sz= 1.025,
    Orientation= [.034,-.009, .999]

Org disp(1.0000000, 1.0181723, .0000000),
    new center is: (82.1723220 78.4665050,-65.0000000).

9). ENTERING Left Kidney
    1). EXITING LKDNY1. Results are: Conf= 1.000,
        Dx= -1.552, Dy= -.262, Dz= .000,
        Dist= 4.894, Scale= 1.816,
    2). EXITING LKDNY2. Results are: Conf= 1.000,
        Dx= -.395, Dy= -.380, Dz= .000,
        Dist= 2.308, Scale= 1.231,

3). EXITING LKDNY3. Results are: Conf= 1.000,
    Dx= .036, Dy= .710, Dz= .000,
    Dist= -.348, Scale= .978,
4). EXITING LKDNY4. Results are: Conf= .810,
    Dx= .342, Dy= .425, Dz= .000,
    Dist= -1.750, Scale= .913,
5). EXITING LKDNY5. Results are: Conf= .773,
    Dx= -.144, Dy= 1.499, Dz= .000,
    Dist= -1.600, Scale= .924,
6). EXITING LKDNY6. Results are: Conf= .810,
    Dx= 1.612, Dy= .597, Dz= .000,
    Dist= -2.429, Scale= .879,
7). EXITING LKDNY7. Results are: Conf= 1.000,
    Dx= .682, Dy= .756, Dz= .000,
    Dist= -1.154, Scale= .928,
8). EXITING LKDNY8. Results are: Conf= 1.000,
    Dx= 2.381, Dy= -.044, Dz= .000,
    Dist= 1.125, Scale= 1.113,
9). EXITING LKDNY9. Results are: Conf= 1.000,
    Dx= -.223, Dy= -.594, Dz= .000,
    Dist= .857, Scale= 1.143,

10). EXITING Zscan of LKDNY1.
    Results are: Conf= 1.000, Zdisp= -1.000,
11). EXITING Zscan of LKDNY9.
    Results are: Conf= .857, Zdisp= 1.000,

9). EXITING Left Kidney.
    Resources: WR= 0, RD= 0,
              CPU= 14.705, RTIME= 58.483,
    Results are: Conf= .929, Dcnf= .000, Dx= .000
    Dz= .000, Dy= .000, Scnf= .929,
    Sx= .976, Sy= .976, Sz= 1.025,
    Orientation= [.032, .003, .999]

Org scale (1.0000000, 1.0000000, 1.0250000),
    new size: (40.000000 40.000000 90.200001).

10). ENTERING Left Kidney
    1). EXITING LKDNY1. Results are: Conf= 1.000,
        Dx= -1.552, Dy= -.262, Dz= .000,
        Dist= 4.894, Scale= 1.816,
    2). EXITING LKDNY2. Results are: Conf= 1.000,
        Dx= -.395, Dy= -.380, Dz= .000,
        Dist= 2.308, Scale= 1.231,
    3). EXITING LKDNY3. Results are: Conf= 1.000,
        Dx= .036, Dy= .710, Dz= .000,
        Dist= -.348, Scale= .978,
    4). EXITING LKDNY4. Results are: Conf= .810,
        Dx= .342, Dy= .425, Dz= .000,
        Dist= -1.750, Scale= .913,
    5). EXITING LKDNY5. Results are: Conf= .773,
        Dx= -.144, Dy= 1.499, Dz= .000,
        Dist= -1.600, Scale= .924,
    6). EXITING LKDNY6. Results are: Conf= .810,
        Dx= 1.612, Dy= .597, Dz= .000,
        Dist= -2.429, Scale= .879,
    7). EXITING LKDNY7. Results are: Conf= 1.000,
        Dx= .682, Dy= .756, Dz= .000,
        Dist= -1.154, Scale= .928,
    8). EXITING LKDNY8. Results are: Conf= 1.000,
        Dx= 2.381, Dy= -.044, Dz= .000,
        Dist= 1.125, Scale= 1.113,
    9). EXITING LKDNY9. Results are: Conf= 1.000,
        Dx= -.223, Dy= -.594, Dz= .000,
        Dist= .857, Scale= 1.143,

    10). EXITING Zscan of LKDNY1.
        Results are: Conf= 1.000, Zdisp= .000,
    11). EXITING Zscan of LKDNY9.
        Results are: Conf= .857, Zdisp= .000,

10). EXITING Left Kidney.
    Resources: WR= 0, RD= 0,
                CPU= 15.800, RTIME= 1:21.433,
    Results are: Conf= .667, Dcnf= .000, Dx= .000,
        Dz= .000, Dy= .000, Scnf= .667,
        Sx= .942, Sy= .942, Sz= 1.000,
        Orientation= [.031, .003, 1.000]

Organ oriented by [.0313421, .0031838, .9995036].

11). ENTERING Left Kidney
   1). EXITING LKDNY1. Results are: Conf= 1.000,
      Dx= -1.936, Dy= -.339, Dz= .062,
      Dist= 4.286, Scale= 1.714,
   2). EXITING LKDNY2. Results are: Conf= 1.000,
      Dx= .270, Dy= -.209, Dz= -.008,
      Dist= 1.188, Scale= 1.119,
   3). EXITING LKDNY3. Results are: Conf= 1.000,
      Dx= .443, Dy= .762, Dz= -.016,
      Dist= -.875, Scale= .945,
   4). EXITING LKDNY4. Results are: Conf= .810,
      Dx= .374, Dy= .384, Dz= -.013,
      Dist= -1.375, Scale= .931,
   5). EXITING LKDNY5. Results are: Conf= .773,
      Dx= .815, Dy= 1.788, Dz= -.031,
      Dist= -3.143, Scale= .850,
   6). EXITING LKDNY6. Results are: Conf= .810,
      Dx= 1.225, Dy= .737, Dz= -.041,
      Dist= -2.333, Scale= .883,
   7). EXITING LKDNY7. Results are: Conf= 1.000,
      Dx= .684, Dy= .818, Dz= -.024,
      Dist= -1.650, Scale= .897,
   8). EXITING LKDNY8. Results are: Conf= 1.000,
      Dx= -.166, Dy= -.225, Dz= .006,
      Dist= .400, Scale= 1.040,
   9). EXITING LKDNY9. Results are: Conf= 1.000,
      Dx= -1.179, Dy= -.359, Dz= .038,
      Dist= .839, Scale= 1.140,

  10). EXITING Zscan of LKDNY1.
      Results are: Conf= 1.000, Zdisp= .000,
  11). EXITING Zscan of LKDNY9.
      Results are: Conf= .714, Zdisp= 2.000,

  11). EXITING Left Kidney.
    Resources: WR= 0, RD= 0,
                CPU= 15.803, RTIME= 1:15.967,
    Results are: Conf= .857, Dcnf= .611, Dx= .575,
        Dz= -.023, Dy= .687, Scnf= .857,
        Sx= .962, Sy= .962, Sz= 1.025,

        Orientation= [.009, .004, 1.000]

Org disp(.0000000, 1.0000000, .0000000),
  new center is: (81.1723220 79.4665050,-65.0000000).

12). ENTERING Left Kidney
   1). EXITING LKDNY1. Results are: Conf= 1.000
      Dx= -.559, Dy= -.696, Dz= .020,
      Dist= 4.542, Scale= 1.757,
   2). EXITING LKDNY2. Results are: Conf= 1.000
      Dx= .939, Dy= -.346, Dz= -.028,
      Dist= 2.076, Scale= 1.208,
   3). EXITING LKDNY3. Results are: Conf= 1.000
      Dx= .236, Dy= .541, Dz= -.009,
      Dist= .176, Scale= 1.011,
   4). EXITING LKDNY4. Results are: Conf= .810
      Dx= .335, Dy= .540, Dz= -.012,
      Dist= -1.600, Scale= .920,
   5). EXITING LKDNY5. Results are: Conf= .773
      Dx= -.017, Dy= .719, Dz= -.002,
      Dist= -2.291, Scale= .891,

   6). EXITING LKDNY6. Results are: Conf= .810
      Dx= 1.023, Dy= .213, Dz= -.033,
      Dist= -2.000, Scale= .900,
   7). EXITING LKDNY7. Results are: Conf= 1.000
      Dx= .532, Dy= .117, Dz= -.017,
      Dist= -1.000, Scale= .938,
   8). EXITING LKDNY8. Results are: Conf= 1.000
      Dx= -.204, Dy= .408, Dz= .005,
      Dist= .989, Scale= 1.099,
   9). EXITING LKDNY9. Results are: Conf= 1.000
      Dx= -1.199, Dy= .012, Dz= .038,
      Dist= 1.243, Scale= 1.207,

  10). EXITING Zscan of LKDNY1.
      Results are: Conf= 1.000, Zdisp= .000,
  11). EXITING Zscan of LKDNY9.
      Results are: Conf= .714, Zdisp= 2.000,

  12). EXITING Left Kidney.
    Resources: WR= 0, RD= 0,
                CPU= 15.959, RTIME= 1:29.133,
    Results are: Conf= .857, Dcnf= .000, Dx= .000,
        Dz= .000, Dy= .000, Scnf= .857,
        Sx= .964, Sy= .964, Sz= 1.025,
        Orientation= [-.002, .006, 1.000]

Org scale (1.0000000, 1.0000000, 1.0250000)
  new size: (40.000000 40.000000 92.455001).

  13). ENTERING LKDNY1- Modifications
   1). EXITING LKDNY1. Results are: Conf= 1.000
      Dx= .548, Dy= .283, Dz= -.018,
      Dist= -1.500, Scale= .750,
  LKDNY1 Distance= -.6000000. scale= .9000000

   2). EXITING LKDNY1. Results are: Conf= 1.000
      Dx= .214, Dy= .007, Dz= -.013,
      Dist= -1.589, Scale= .706,
  LKDNY1 Distance= -.5400000. scale= .9000000

   3). EXITING LKDNY1. Results are: Conf= 1.000
      Dx= .556, Dy= -.168, Dz= -.051,
      Dist= -2.299, Scale= .527,
  LKDNY1 disp= (.5561671, .0000000)= .5561671
  New center= [.5561671, .0000000].

   4). EXITING LKDNY1. Results are: Conf= 1.000
      Dx= .098, Dy= .312, Dz= -.016,
      Dist= .809, Scale= 1.166,
  LKDNY1 Distance= .4860000. scale= 1.1000000

   5). EXITING LKDNY1. Results are: Conf= 1.000
      Dx= -1.207, Dy= .891, Dz= .176,
      Dist= 2.633, Scale= 1.493,
  LKDNY1 Distance= .5346000. scale= 1.1000000

   6). EXITING LKDNY1. Results are: Conf= 1.000
      Dx= -1.196, Dy= -.102, Dz= .230,
      Dist= .667, Scale= 1.113,
  LKDNY1 Distance= .5880600. scale= 1.1000000

   7). EXITING LKDNY1. Results are: Conf= 1.000
      Dx= -1.156, Dy= 1.041, Dz= .234,
      Dist= .987, Scale= 1.153,
  LKDNY1 No changes

   13). EXITING LKDNY1- Modifications.
      Resources: WR= 0, RD= 0,
            CPU= 5.415, RTIME= 26.533,

14). ENTERING LKDNY2- Modifications
   1). EXITING LKDNY2. Results are: Conf= 1.000
      Dx= .939, Dy= -.346, Dz= -.028,
      Dist= 2.076, Scale= 1.208,
LKDNY2 Distance= .9999999. scale= 1.1000000

   2). EXITING LKDNY2. Results are: Conf= 1.000
      Dx= -.189, Dy= -.073, Dz= .012,
      Dist= .780, Scale= 1.071,
LKDNY2 Distance= .7804877. scale= 1.0709534

   3). EXITING LKDNY2. Results are: Conf= 1.000
      Dx= .411, Dy= -.486, Dz= -.034,
      Dist= .462, Scale= 1.039,
LKDNY2 disp= (.4108517, .0000000)= .4108517
     New center= [.4108517, .0000000].

   4). EXITING LKDNY2. Results are: Conf= 1.000
      Dx= .241, Dy= -.270, Dz= -.027,
      Dist= .385, Scale= 1.033,
LKDNY2 Distance= .3846155. scale= 1.0326485

   5). EXITING LKDNY2. Results are: Conf= 1.000
      Dx= .187, Dy= -.125, Dz= -.027,
      Dist= -.533, Scale= .956,
LKDNY2 No changes

  14). EXITING LKDNY2- Modifications.
    Resources: WR= 0, RD= 0,
           CPU= 7.402, RTIME= 37.200,

  15). ENTERING LKDNY3- Modifications
   1). EXITING LKDNY3. Results are: Conf= 1.000
      Dx= .014, Dy= .488, Dz= -.002,
      Dist= -.111, Scale= .993,
LKDNY3 disp= (.0137597, .4881916)= .4883855
     New center= [.0137597, .4881916].

   2). EXITING LKDNY3. Results are: Conf= 1.000
      Dx= .282, Dy= .514, Dz= -.021,
      Dist= -.067, Scale= .996,
LKDNY3 disp= (.2817502, .5139695)= .5861295
     New center= [.2955099, 1.0021611].

   3). EXITING LKDNY3. Results are: Conf= 1.000
      Dx= .501, Dy= .378, Dz= -.051,
      Dist= .692, Scale= 1.043,
LKDNY3 disp= (.5008594, .3776318)= .6272687
     New center= [.7963693, 1.3797929].

   4). EXITING LKDNY3. Results are: Conf= 1.000
      Dx= .149, Dy= .248, Dz= -.022,
      Dist= -.091, Scale= .994,
LKDNY3 No changes

  15). EXITING LKDNY3- Modifications.
    Resources: WR= 1, RD= 0,
           CPU= 6.78, RTIME= 21.0,

  16). ENTERING LKDNY4- Modifications
   1). EXITING LKDNY4. Results are: Conf= .810
      Dx= .335, Dy= .540, Dz= -.012,
      Dist= -1.600, Scale= .920,
LKDNY4 Distance= -1.6000000. scale= .9200000

   2). EXITING LKDNY4. Results are: Conf= .789
      Dx= -.337, Dy= .261, Dz= .019,
      Dist= -.000, Scale= 1.000,
LKDNY4 disp= (-.3370195, .2607975)= .4261425
     New center= [-.3370195, .2607975].

   3). EXITING LKDNY4. Results are: Conf= .789
      Dx= -.669, Dy= .077, Dz= .062,
      Dist= -.111, Scale= .994,
LKDNY4 No changes

  16). EXITING LKDNY4- Modifications.
    Resources: WR= 0, RD= 0,
           CPU= 7.280, RTIME= 31.200,

  17). ENTERING LKDNY5- Modifications
   1). EXITING LKDNY5. Results are: Conf= .773
      Dx= -.017, Dy= .719, Dz= -.002,
      Dist= -2.291, Scale= .891,
LKDNY5 Distance= -2.1000000. scale= .9000000

   2). EXITING LKDNY5. Results are: Conf= .800
      Dx= -.406, Dy= 1.027, Dz= .019,
      Dist= -.600, Scale= .968,
LKDNY5 disp= (-.4056364, 1.0265880)= 1.1038224
     New center= [-.4056364, 1.0265880].

   3). EXITING LKDNY5. Results are: Conf= .800
      Dx= -.106, Dy= .260, Dz= .008,
      Dist= -.629, Scale= .967,
LKDNY5 No changes

  17). EXITING LKDNY5- Modifications.
    Resources: WR= 0, RD= 0,
           CPU= 6.256, RTIME= 24.83,

  18). ENTERING LKDNY6- Modifications
   1). EXITING LKDNY6. Results are: Conf= .810
      Dx= 1.023, Dy= .213, Dz= -.033,
      Dist= -2.000, Scale= .900,
LKDNY6 disp= (1.0228422, .2134938)= 1.0448855
     New center= [1.0228422, .2134938].

   2). EXITING LKDNY6. Results are: Conf= .810
      Dx= .701, Dy= .190, Dz= -.045,
      Dist= -1.727, Scale= .914,
LKDNY6 Distance= -1.7272727. scale= .9136364

   3). EXITING LKDNY6. Results are: Conf= .789
      Dx= .047, Dy= .252, Dz= -.007,
      Dist= -.429, Scale= .977,
LKDNY6 No changes

  18). EXITING LKDNY6- Modifications.
    Resources: WR= 0, RD= 0,
           CPU= 6.6, RTIME= 21.83,

  19). ENTERING LKDNY7- Modifications
   1). EXITING LKDNY7. Results are: Conf= 1.000
      Dx= .532, Dy= .117, Dz= -.017,
      Dist= -1.000, Scale= .938,
LKDNY7 disp= (.5317965, .1170661)= .5445291
     New center= [.5317965, .1170661].

   2). EXITING LKDNY7. Results are: Conf= 1.000
      Dx= .821, Dy= .246, Dz= -.053,
      Dist= .200, Scale= 1.013,
LKDNY7 disp= (.8212591, .2455173)= .8571728
     New center= [1.3530555, .3625833].

   3). EXITING LKDNY7. Results are: Conf= 1.000
      Dx= .919, Dy= -.256, Dz= -.084,
      Dist= -.048, Scale= .997,
LKDNY7 disp= (.9194853, .0000000)= .9194853
     New center= [2.2725408, .3625833].

   4). EXITING LKDNY7. Results are: Conf= .941

```
          Dx= .420, Dy= -.007, Dz= -.053,
          Dist= .316, Scale= 1.020,
LKDNY7 disp= ( .4201407, .0000000)= .4201407
   New center= [ 2.6926815, .3625833].

   5). EXITING LKDNY7. Results are: Conf= 1.000
          Dx= .354, Dy= .390, Dz= -.062,
          Dist= 1.387, Scale= 1.087,
LKDNY7 Distance= 1.3870969. scale= 1.0866936

   6). EXITING LKDNY7. Results are: Conf= 1.000
          Dx= 1.087, Dy= 1.130, Dz= -.229,
          Dist= .706, Scale= 1.041,
LKDNY7 disp= ( 1.0870052, .0000000)= 1.0870052
   New center= [ 3.7796866, .3625833].

   7). EXITING LKDNY7. Results are: Conf= 1.000
          Dx= .292, Dy= .457, Dz= -.075,
          Dist= 1.176, Scale= 1.068,
LKDNY7 Distance= 1.1764706. scale= 1.0676634

   8). EXITING LKDNY7. Results are: Conf= 1.000
          Dx= .619, Dy= .585, Dz= -.174,
          Dist= -.762, Scale= .959,
LKDNY7 disp= ( .6187332, .5854671)= .8518231
   New center= [ 4.3984199, .9480505].

   9). EXITING LKDNY7. Results are: Conf= 1.000
          Dx= .425, Dy= .327, Dz= -.133,
          Dist= -.485, Scale= .974,
LKDNY7 disp= ( .4250445, .3268214)= .5361670
   New center= [ 4.8234643, 1.2748719].

   10). EXITING LKDNY7. Results are: Conf= 1.000
          Dx= -.029, Dy= .443, Dz= -.005,
          Dist= .091, Scale= 1.005,
LKDNY7 disp= ( .0000000, .4431074)= .4431074
   New center= [ 4.8234643, 1.7179793].

   11). EXITING LKDNY7. Results are: Conf= 1.000
          Dx= .343, Dy= -.284, Dz= -.113,
          Dist= -.316, Scale= .983,
LKDNY7 disp= ( .3434456, .0000000)= .3434456
   New center= [ 5.1669099, 1.7179793].

   19). EXITING LKDNY7- Modifications.
          Resources: WR= 0, RD= 0,
                CPU= 20.912, RTIME= 1:35.284,

   20). ENTERING LKDNY8- Modifications
   1). EXITING LKDNY8. Results are: Conf= 1.000
          Dx= -.260, Dy= .207, Dz= .007,
          Dist= 1.902, Scale= 1.190,
LKDNY8 Distance= .9999999. scale= 1.1000000

   2). EXITING LKDNY8. Results are: Conf= 1.000
          Dx= .276, Dy= -.586, Dz= -.014,
          Dist= 1.300, Scale= 1.118,
LKDNY8 Distance= 1.0999999. scale= 1.1000000

   3). EXITING LKDNY8. Results are: Conf= 1.000
          Dx= .560, Dy= -.723, Dz= -.046,
          Dist= .500, Scale= 1.041,
LKDNY8 disp= ( .5595863, .0000000)= .5595863
   New center= [ .5595863, .0000000].

   4). EXITING LKDNY8. Results are: Conf= 1.000
          Dx= 1.562, Dy= -.734, Dz= -.187,
          Dist= .583, Scale= 1.048,
LKDNY8 disp= ( .8347584, .0000000)= .8347584
   New center= [ 1.3943447, .0000000].
```

```
   5). EXITING LKDNY8. Results are: Conf= 1.000
          Dx= 1.178, Dy= .171, Dz= -.189,
          Dist= 1.417, Scale= 1.117,
LKDNY8 disp= ( .8347584, .1709430)= .8520816
   New center= [ 2.2291031, .1709430].

   6). EXITING LKDNY8. Results are: Conf= 1.000
          Dx= .956, Dy= -.216, Dz= -.178,
          Dist= 2.467, Scale= 1.204,
LKDNY8 Distance= 1.2099999. scale= 1.1000000

   7). EXITING LKDNY8. Results are: Conf= 1.000
          Dx= .729, Dy= -.154, Dz= -.159,
          Dist= .125, Scale= 1.009,
LKDNY8 disp= ( .7286755, .0000000)= .7286755
   New center= [ 2.9577786, .1709430].

   8). EXITING LKDNY8. Results are: Conf= 1.000
          Dx= 2.337, Dy= .244, Dz= -.605,
          Dist= 1.333, Scale= 1.100,
LKDNY8 disp= ( .8347584, .2436191)= .8695814
   New center= [ 3.7925370, .4145620].

   9). EXITING LKDNY8. Results are: Conf= 1.000
          Dx= .835, Dy= -.393, Dz= -.231,
          Dist= 1.692, Scale= 1.127,
LKDNY8 Distance= 1.3309999. scale= 1.1000000

   10). EXITING LKDNY8. Results are: Conf= 1.000
          Dx= 1.033, Dy= .077, Dz= -.338,
          Dist= .900, Scale= 1.061,
LKDNY8 disp= ( .8347584, .0000000)= .8347584
   New center= [ 4.6272954, .4145620].

   11). EXITING LKDNY8. Results are: Conf= 1.000
          Dx= .407, Dy= .490, Dz= -.164,
          Dist= .755, Scale= 1.052,
LKDNY8 disp= ( .4066896, .0000000)= .4066896
   New center= [ 5.0339850, .4145620].

   20). EXITING LKDNY8- Modifications.
          Resources: WR= 1, RD= 0,
                CPU= 17.387, RTIME= 1:27.216,

   21). ENTERING LKDNY9- Modifications
   1). EXITING LKDNY9. Results are: Conf= .857
          Dx= 2.684, Dy= .779, Dz= -.087,
          Dist= -1.063, Scale= .823,
LKDNY9 disp= ( .8347584, .7792178)= 1.1419290
   New center= [ .8347584, .7792178].

   2). EXITING LKDNY9. Results are: Conf= 1.000
          Dx= 2.046, Dy= 1.256, Dz= -.136,
          Dist= -.750, Scale= .875,
LKDNY9 disp= ( .8347584, .8347584)= 1.1805266
   New center= [ 1.6695168, 1.6139762].

   3). EXITING LKDNY9. Results are: Conf= .857
          Dx= .833, Dy= .038, Dz= -.079,
          Dist= -1.200, Scale= .800,
LKDNY9 disp= ( .8327440, .0384741)= .8336323
   New center= [ 2.5022608, 1.6524503].

   4). EXITING LKDNY9. Results are: Conf= 1.000
          Dx= 1.238, Dy= .032, Dz= -.156,
          Dist= -1.000, Scale= .833,
LKDNY9 disp= ( .8347584, .0317197)= .8353608
   New center= [ 3.3370192, 1.6841700].

   5). EXITING LKDNY9. Results are: Conf= 1.000
          Dx= -.724, Dy= .189, Dz= .111,
          Dist= .818, Scale= 1.136,
LKDNY9 Distance= .6000000. scale= 1.1000000
```

6). EXITING LKDNY9. Results are: Conf= 1.000
       Dx= .089, Dy= .538, Dz= -.027,
       Dist= .889, Scale= 1.135,
LKDNY9 disp= (.0886048, .5377481)= .5449990
    New center= [3.4256240, 2.2219181].
7). EXITING LKDNY9. Results are: Conf= 1.000
       Dx= .067, Dy= .214, Dz= -.020,
       Dist= -.432, Scale= .934,
LKDNY9 No changes

21). EXITING LKDNY9- Modifications.
     Resources: WR= 0, RD= 0,
                     CPU= 6.670, RTIME= 29.83,

22). ENTERING Left Kidney
    1). EXITING LKDNY1. Results are: Conf= 1.000
           Dx= .478, Dy= 1.027, Dz= -.006,
           Dist= -2.516, Scale= .611,
    2). EXITING LKDNY2. Results are: Conf= 1.000
           Dx= .223, Dy= -.079, Dz= -.004,
           Dist= -.786, Scale= .935,
    3). EXITING LKDNY3. Results are: Conf= 1.000
           Dx= .187, Dy= .298, Dz= -.004,
           Dist= .500, Scale= 1.031,
    4). EXITING LKDNY4. Results are: Conf= .789
           Dx= -.143, Dy= .150, Dz= -.001,
           Dist= -.643, Scale= .965,
    5). EXITING LKDNY5. Results are: Conf= .800
           Dx= -.106, Dy= .260, Dz= .009,
           Dist= -.629, Scale= .967,
    6). EXITING LKDNY6. Results are: Conf= .789
           Dx= -.097, Dy= .027, Dz= .026,
           Dist= .200, Scale= 1.011,
    7). EXITING LKDNY7. Results are: Conf= 1.000
           Dx= .407, Dy= -.198, Dz= -.082,
           Dist= -.571, Scale= .969,
    8). EXITING LKDNY8. Results are: Conf= 1.000
           Dx= .589, Dy= .511, Dz= .024,
           Dist= .500, Scale= 1.034,
    9). EXITING LKDNY9. Results are: Conf= .857
           Dx= -.405, Dy= 1.557, Dz= -.587,
           Dist= 3.889, Scale= 1.589,

    10). EXITING Zscan of LKDNY1.
           Results are: Conf= 1.000, Zdisp= 1.000,
    11). EXITING Zscan of LKDNY9.
           Results are: Conf= .714, Zdisp= 8.556,

22). EXITING Left Kidney.
     Resources: WR= 0, RD= 114,
                     CPU= 18.856, RTIME= 57.234,
     Results are: Conf= .857, Dcnf= .857, Dx= .000,
       Dz= 4.778, Dy= .000, Scnf= .000,
       Sx= 1.000, Sy= 1.000, Sz= 1.000,
       Orientation= [-.002, .003, 1.000]

Org disp(.0000000, .0000000, 4.7777777),
  new center is: (82.1723220, 79.4665050,-60.2222220).

23). ENTERING Left Kidney
    1). EXITING LKDNY1. Results are: Conf= 1.000
           Dx= -1.889, Dy= -1.493, Dz= .016,
           Dist= 4.729, Scale= 1.731,
    2). EXITING LKDNY2. Results are: Conf= 1.000
           Dx= -.194, Dy= -.785, Dz= .074,
           Dist= 1.769, Scale= 1.145,
    3). EXITING LKDNY3. Results are: Conf= 1.000
           Dx= -.572, Dy= -.053, Dz= .000,
           Dist= 2.846, Scale= 1.178,
    4). EXITING LKDNY4. Results are: Conf= .789
           Dx= -.605, Dy= .114, Dz= -.011,
           Dist= .320, Scale= 1.017,

    5). EXITING LKDNY5. Results are: Conf= .800
           Dx= .249, Dy= -.174, Dz= -.022,
           Dist= -.273, Scale= .986,
    6). EXITING LKDNY6. Results are: Conf= .789
           Dx= .338, Dy= .270, Dz= -.102,
           Dist= -.833, Scale= .954,
    7). EXITING LKDNY7. Results are: Conf= 1.000
           Dx= 1.386, Dy= .239, Dz= -.288,
           Dist= -1.405, Scale= .924,
    8). EXITING LKDNY8. Results are: Conf= 1.000
           Dx= .387, Dy= .827, Dz= .000,
           Dist= .300, Scale= 1.020,
    9). EXITING LKDNY9. Results are: Conf= .857
           Dx= 1.174, Dy= .553, Dz= .114,
           Dist= .250, Scale= 1.038,

    10). EXITING Zscan of LKDNY1.
           Results are: Conf= 1.000, Zdisp= -4.000,
    11). EXITING Zscan of LKDNY9.
           Results are: Conf= .714, Zdisp= 4.600,

23). EXITING Left Kidney.
     Resources: WR= 0, RD= 168,
                     CPU= 18.807, RTIME= 58.283,
     Results are: Conf= .857, Dcnf= .000, Dx= .000,
       Dz= .000, Dy= .000, Scnf= .000,
       Sx= 1.000, Sy= 1.000, Sz= 1.100,
       Orientation= [.029, .020, .999]
Org scale (1.0000000, 1.0000000, 1.1000000)
new size: (40.000000 40.000000 101.70050).

24). ENTERING Left Kidney
    1). EXITING LKDNY1. Results are: Conf= 1.000
           Dx= -1.842, Dy= -1.408, Dz= .020,
           Dist= 4.849, Scale= 1.750,
    2). EXITING LKDNY2. Results are: Conf= 1.000
           Dx= .527, Dy= -.197, Dz= -.008,
           Dist= -.867, Scale= .929,
    3). EXITING LKDNY3. Results are: Conf= 1.000
           Dx= -.111, Dy= .414, Dz= -.005,
           Dist= .667, Scale= 1.042,
    4). EXITING LKDNY4. Results are: Conf= .789
           Dx= -.605, Dy= .188, Dz= -.008,
           Dist= .320, Scale= 1.017,
    5). EXITING LKDNY5. Results are: Conf= .800
           Dx= .250, Dy= -.174, Dz= -.021,
           Dist= -.273, Scale= .986,
    6). EXITING LKDNY6. Results are: Conf= .789
           Dx= 1.072, Dy= .103, Dz= -.274,
           Dist= -1.727, Scale= .905,
    7). EXITING LKDNY7. Results are: Conf= 1.000
           Dx= 1.590, Dy= 1.113, Dz= -.315,
           Dist= -2.091, Scale= .887,
    8). EXITING LKDNY8. Results are: Conf= 1.000
           Dx= 3.308, Dy= 1.672, Dz= .148,
           Dist= -1.250, Scale= .915,
    9). EXITING LKDNY9. Results are: Conf= 1.000
           Dx= .396, Dy= .448, Dz= -.041,
           Dist= -1.571, Scale= .762,

    10). EXITING Zscan of LKDNY1.
           Results are: Conf= 1.000, Zdisp= .000,
    11). EXITING Zscan of LKDNY9.
           Results are: Conf= .714, Zdisp= .400,

24). EXITING Left Kidney.
     Resources: WR= 0, RD= 429,
                     CPU= 23.290, RTIME= 1:32.816,
     Results are: Conf= .000, Dcnf= .000, Dx= .000,
       Dz= .000, Dy= .000, Scnf= .000,
       Sx= 1.000, Sy= 1.000, Sz= 1.000,
       Orientation= [.034, .020, .999]

Organ oriented by [.0341039, .0198153, .9992218].

25). ENTERING Left Kidney
  1). EXITING LKDNY1. Results are: Conf= 1.000,
    Dx= -.034, Dy= .134, Dz= -.002,
    Dist= 1.714, Scale= 1.265,
  2). EXITING LKDNY2. Results are: Conf= 1.000,
    Dx= .509, Dy= .170, Dz= -.056,
    Dist= .500, Scale= 1.041,
  3). EXITING LKDNY3. Results are: Conf= 1.000,
    Dx= .414, Dy= .301, Dz= -.025,
    Dist= -.632, Scale= .961,
  4). EXITING LKDNY4. Results are: Conf= .789,
    Dx= -.324, Dy= .180, Dz= .004,
    Dist= .200, Scale= 1.011,
  5). EXITING LKDNY5. Results are: Conf= .800,
    Dx= .360, Dy= -.070, Dz= -.041,
    Dist= -.333, Scale= .982,
  6). EXITING LKDNY6. Results are: Conf= .789,
    Dx= .649, Dy= .437, Dz= -.210,
    Dist= -1.182, Scale= .935,
  7). EXITING LKDNY7. Results are: Conf= 1.000,
    Dx= 1.405, Dy= .819, Dz= -.343,
    Dist= -1.971, Scale= .894,
  8). EXITING LKDNY8. Results are: Conf= 1.000,
    Dx= 2.129, Dy= 1.291, Dz= -.009,
    Dist= -.667, Scale= .954,
  9). EXITING LKDNY9. Results are: Conf= 1.000,
    Dx= .208, Dy= .941, Dz= -.248,
    Dist= .473, Scale= 1.072,

  10). EXITING Zscan of LKDNY1.
    Results are: Conf= .857, Zdisp= .000,
  11). EXITING Zscan of LKDNY9.
    Results are: Conf= .857, Zdisp= .800,

25). EXITING Left Kidney.
  Resources: WR= 0, RD= 474,
        CPU= 24.789, RTIME= 1:42.750,
  Results are: Conf= .000, Dcnf= .000, Dx= .000,
  Dz= .000, Dy= .000, Scnf= .000,
  Sx= 1.000, Sy= 1.000, Sz= 1.000,
  Orientation= [.015, .013, 1.000]

Organ oriented by [.0153530, .0126353, .9998023].

26). ENTERING Left Kidney
  1). EXITING LKDNY1. Results are: Conf= 1.000,
    Dx= -1.005, Dy= -.804, Dz= .087,
    Dist= 2.286, Scale= 1.353,
  2). EXITING LKDNY2. Results are: Conf= 1.000,
    Dx= .411, Dy= .390, Dz= -.081,
    Dist= -.350, Scale= .971,
  3). EXITING LKDNY3. Results are: Conf= 1.000,
    Dx= -.378, Dy= .277, Dz= .007,
    Dist= 1.833, Scale= 1.115,
  4). EXITING LKDNY4. Results are: Conf= .789,
    Dx= -.308, Dy= .365, Dz= .002,
    Dist= .360, Scale= 1.020,
  5). EXITING LKDNY5. Results are: Conf= .800,
    Dx= .215, Dy= .009, Dz= -.029,
    Dist= -.429, Scale= .977,
  6). EXITING LKDNY6. Results are: Conf= .789,
    Dx= .328, Dy= .610, Dz= -.139,
    Dist= -1.000, Scale= .945,
  7). EXITING LKDNY7. Results are: Conf= 1.000,
    Dx= .759, Dy= .975, Dz= -.227,
    Dist= -1.114, Scale= .940,
  8). EXITING LKDNY8. Results are: Conf= 1.000,
    Dx= .368, Dy= 1.600, Dz= -.095,
    Dist= .368, Scale= 1.025,

  9). EXITING LKDNY9. Results are: Conf= 1.000,
    Dx= .692, Dy= 1.389, Dz= -.324,
    Dist= -2.400, Scale= .636,

  10). EXITING Zscan of LKDNY1.
    Results are: Conf= .857, Zdisp= .000,
  11). EXITING Zscan of LKDNY9.
    Results are: Conf= .714, Zdisp= 2.250,

26). EXITING Left Kidney.
  Resources: WR= 0, RD= 13,
        CPU= 17.339, RTIME= 51.434,
  Results are: Conf= .786, Dcnf= .000, Dx= .000,
  Dz= .000, Dy= .000, Scnf= .786,
  Sx= 1.000, Sy= 1.000, Sz= 1.028,
  Orientation= [.014, .021, 1.000]

Org scale (1.0000000, 1.0000000, 1.0281250)
  new size: (40.000000 40.000000 104.56083).

  27). **ENTERING Left Kidney**
    1). EXITING LKDNY1. Results are: Conf= 1.000,
      Dx= 1.942, Dy= 1.125, Dz= -.154,
      Dist= -3.702, Scale= .428,
    2). EXITING LKDNY2. Results are: Conf= 1.000,
      Dx= 1.043, Dy= .545, Dz= -.156,
      Dist= -.454, Scale= .963,
    3). EXITING LKDNY3. Results are: Conf= 1.000,
      Dx= .535, Dy= .429, Dz= -.048,
      Dist= -.667, Scale= .958,
    4). EXITING LKDNY4. Results are: Conf= .789,
      Dx= -.308, Dy= .365, Dz= .003,
      Dist= .360, Scale= 1.020,
    5). EXITING LKDNY5. Results are: Conf= .800,
      Dx= .215, Dy= .009, Dz= -.029,
      Dist= -.429, Scale= .977,
    6). EXITING LKDNY6. Results are: Conf= .789,
      Dx= .329, Dy= .610, Dz= -.137,
      Dist= -1.000, Scale= .945,
    7). EXITING LKDNY7. Results are: Conf= 1.000,
      Dx= 1.183, Dy= .861, Dz= -.319,
      Dist= -1.571, Scale= .915,
    8). EXITING LKDNY8. Results are: Conf= 1.000,
      Dx= 1.809, Dy= 1.328, Dz= -.067,
      Dist= 1.000, Scale= 1.068,
    9). EXITING LKDNY9. Results are: Conf= .857,
      Dz= 2.494, Dy= 1.769, Dz= -.140,
      Dist= -3.360, Scale= .491,

    10). EXITING Zscan of LKDNY1.
      Results are: Conf= .857, Zdisp= .909,
    11). EXITING Zscan of LKDNY9.
      Results are: Conf= .857, Zdisp= -.333,

  27). EXITING Left Kidney.
    Resources: WR= 0, RD= 83,
          CPU= 18.890, RTIME= 59.533,
    Results are: Conf= .857, Dcnf= .000, Dx= .000,
    Dz= .000, Dy= .000, Scnf= .857,
    Sx= .984, Sy= .984, Sz= .984,
    Orientation= [.010, .011, 1.000]

Organ - No changes

  28). ENTERING LKDNY1- Modifications
    1). EXITING LKDNY1. Results are: Conf= 1.000,
      Dx= 1.942, Dy= 1.125, Dz= -.154,
      Dist= -3.702, Scale= .428,
LKDNY1 Distance= -.6468660. scale= .9000000

2). EXITING LKDNY1. Results are: Conf= 1.000,
    Dx= .666, Dy= .833, Dz= -.153,
    Dist= -.218, Scale= .963,
LKDNY1 disp= (.6660952, .7327701)= .9902701
    New center= [1.2222624, .7327701].

3). EXITING LKDNY1. Results are: Conf= 1.000,
    Dx= .909, Dy= 1.235, Dz= -.339,
    Dist= -1.026, Scale= .824,
LKDNY1 disp= (.7327701, .7327701)= 1.0362934
    New center= [1.9550325, 1.4655402].

4). EXITING LKDNY1. Results are: Conf= 1.000,
    Dx= .343, Dy= .222, Dz= -.140,
    Dist= -1.000, Scale= .828,
LKDNY1 disp= (.3425982, .2223728)= .4084400
    New center= [2.2976307, 1.6879131].

5). EXITING LKDNY1. Results are: Conf= 1.000,
    Dx= .557, Dy= 1.819, Dz= -.572,
    Dist= -1.289, Scale= .779,
LKDNY1 disp= (.5574229, .7327701)= .9206913
    New center= [2.8550536, 2.4206832].

6). EXITING LKDNY1. Results are: Conf= 1.000,
    Dx= .067, Dy= -.117, Dz= -.006,
    Dist= 1.000, Scale= 1.172,
LKDNY1 Distance= .5821794. scale= 1.1000000

7). EXITING LKDNY1. Results are: Conf= 1.000,
    Dx= -1.039, Dy= .438, Dz= .519,
    Dist= .823, Scale= 1.128,
LKDNY1 disp= (.0000000, .4378449)= .4378449
    New center= [2.8550536, 2.8585281].

8). EXITING LKDNY1. Results are: Conf= 1.000,
    Dx= -1.596, Dy= -.716, Dz= 1.433,
    Dist= 3.368, Scale= 1.526,
LKDNY1 Distance= .6403973. scale= 1.1000000

9). EXITING LKDNY1. Results are: Conf= 1.000,
    Dx= -1.245, Dy= .320, Dz= .979,
    Dist= 2.697, Scale= 1.383,
LKDNY1 Distance= .7044370. scale= 1.1000000

10). EXITING LKDNY1. Results are: Conf= 1.000,
    Dx= -.953, Dy= .429, Dz= .806,
    Dist= 1.868, Scale= 1.241,
LKDNY1 Distance= .7748807. scale= 1.1000000

11). EXITING LKDNY1. Results are: Conf= 1.000,
    Dx= -.332, Dy= -.470, Dz= .697,
    Dist= -1.383, Scale= .838,
LKDNY1 No changes

28). EXITING LKDNY1- Modifications.
    Resources: WR= 1, RD= 19,
          CPU= 9.511, RTIME= 51.50,

29). ENTERING LKDNY2- Modifications
  1). EXITING LKDNY2. Results are: Conf= 1.000,
    Dx= 1.043, Dy= .545, Dz= -.156,
    Dist= -.454, Scale= .963,
LKDNY2 disp= (1.0234010, .5446183)= 1.1592923
    New center= [1.4342527, .5446183].

2). EXITING LKDNY2. Results are: Conf= 1.000,
    Dx= .451, Dy= .361, Dz= -.132,
    Dist= .462, Scale= 1.038,
LKDNY2 disp= (.4508168, .3607186)= .5773679
    New center= [1.8850695, .9053369].

3). EXITING LKDNY2. Results are: Conf= 1.000,
    Dx= .201, Dy= -.117, Dz= -.031,
    Dist= 1.556, Scale= 1.128,
LKDNY2 Distance= 1.2165103. scale= 1.1000000

4). EXITING LKDNY2. Results are: Conf= 1.000,
    Dx= .595, Dy= -.244, Dz= -.155,
    Dist= -.182, Scale= .986,
LKDNY2 disp= (.5949640, .0000000)= .5949640
    New center= [2.4800335, .9053369].

5). EXITING LKDNY2. Results are: Conf= 1.000,
    Dx= -.708, Dy= -.223, Dz= .380,
    Dist= -.444, Scale= .967,
LKDNY2 No changes

29). EXITING LKDNY2- Modifications.
    Resources: WR= 0, RD= 0,
          CPU= 8.846, RTIME= 27.117,

30). ENTERING LKDNY3- Modifications
  1). EXITING LKDNY3. Results are: Conf= 1.000,
    Dx= .535, Dy= .429, Dz= -.048,
    Dist= -.667, Scale= .958,
LKDNY3 disp= (.5351085, .4291685)= .6859495
    New center= [1.3314779, 1.8089614].

2). EXITING LKDNY3. Results are: Conf= 1.000,
    Dx= -.336, Dy= -.229, Dz= .064,
    Dist= 1.714, Scale= 1.107,
LKDNY3 Distance= 1.5999999. scale= 1.1000000

3). EXITING LKDNY3. Results are: Conf= 1.000,
    Dx= -.883, Dy= -.016, Dz= .194,
    Dist= 1.143, Scale= 1.065,
LKDNY3 Distance= 1.1428570. scale= 1.0649351

4). EXITING LKDNY3. Results are: Conf= 1.000,
    Dx= -.923, Dy= .499, Dz= .203,
    Dist= .000, Scale= 1.000,
LKDNY3 disp= (.0000000, .4988123)= .4988123
    New center= [1.3314779, 2.3077737].

5). EXITING LKDNY3. Results are: Conf= 1.000,
    Dx= -1.015, Dy= .071, Dz= .391,
    Dist= .105, Scale= 1.006,
LKDNY3 No changes

30). EXITING LKDNY3- Modifications.
    Resources: WR= 0, RD= 0,
          CPU= 10.192, RTIME= 27.866,

31). ENTERING LKDNY4- Modifications
  1). EXITING LKDNY4. Results are: Conf= .789,
    Dx= -.308, Dy= .365, Dz= .003,
    Dist= .360, Scale= 1.020,
LKDNY4 disp= (-.3078241, .3647829)= .4773072
    New center= [-.6448435, .6255803].

2). EXITING LKDNY4. Results are: Conf= .737,
    Dx= -.331, Dy= .181, Dz= .028,
    Dist= .500, Scale= 1.027,
LKDNY4 disp= (-.3312622, .1814808)= .3777167
    New center= [-.9761057, .8070611].

3). EXITING LKDNY4. Results are: Conf= .789,
    Dx= -.279, Dy= .213, Dz= .035,
    Dist= .231, Scale= 1.013,
LKDNY4 No changes

31). EXITING LKDNY4- Modifications.
   Resources: WR= 0, RD= 0,
         CPU= 5.979, RTIME= 15.150.

32). ENTERING LKDNY5- Modifications
   1). EXITING LKDNY5. Results are: Conf= .800,
      Dx= .215, Dy= .009, Dz= -.029,
      Dist= -.429, Scale= .977,
LKDNY5 Distance= -.4285714. scale= .9773243

   2). EXITING LKDNY5. Results are: Conf= .789,
      Dx= .077, Dy= -.218, Dz= -.001,
      Dist= .333, Scale= 1.018,
LKDNY5 Distance= .3333333. scale= 1.0180459

   3). EXITING LKDNY5. Results are: Conf= .800,
      Dx= .023, Dy= .001, Dz= -.007,
      Dist= .000, Scale= 1.000,
LKDNY5 No changes

32). EXITING LKDNY5- Modifications.
   Resources: WR= 0, RD= 0,
         CPU= 6.489, RTIME= 18.117,

33). ENTERING LKDNY6- Modifications
   1). EXITING LKDNY6. Results are: Conf= .789,
      Dx= .329, Dy= .610, Dz= -.137,
      Dist= -1.000, Scale= .945,
LKDNY6 disp= (.3286072, .6100989)= .6929671
   New center= [1.3514494, .8235927].

   2). EXITING LKDNY6. Results are: Conf= .789,
      Dx= .550, Dy= -.005, Dz= -.215,
      Dist= -.857, Scale= .953,
LKDNY6 disp= (.5497231, .0000000)= .5497231
   New center= [1.9011725, .8235927].

   3). EXITING LKDNY6. Results are: Conf= .789,
      Dx= .428, Dy= -.170, Dz= -.186,
      Dist= -1.385, Scale= .924,
LKDNY6 disp= (.4280143, .0000000)= .4280143
   New center= [2.3291867, .8235927].
   4). EXITING LKDNY6. Results are: Conf= .789,
      Dx= .193, Dy= .163, Dz= -.146,
      Dist= .118, Scale= 1.006,
LKDNY6 No changes

33). EXITING LKDNY6- Modifications.
   Resources: WR= 1, RD= 0,
         CPU= 9.499, RTIME= 32.633,

34). ENTERING LKDNY7- Modifications
   1). EXITING LKDNY7. Results are: Conf= 1.000,
      Dx= 1.183, Dy= .861, Dz= -.319,
      Dist= -1.571, Scale= .915,
LKDNY7 Distance= -1.5714286. scale= .9153488

   2). EXITING LKDNY7. Results are: Conf= 1.000,
      Dx= 1.230, Dy= .330, Dz= -.427,
      Dist= -.424, Scale= .975,
LKDNY7 Distance= -.4242425. scale= .9750330

   3). EXITING LKDNY7. Results are: Conf= 1.000,
      Dx= .164, Dy= .135, Dz= -.085,
      Dist= .724, Scale= 1.044,
LKDNY7 Distance= .7241380. scale= 1.0437073

   4). EXITING LKDNY7. Results are: Conf= 1.000,
      Dx= .960, Dy= .120, Dz= -.518,
      Dist= -.308, Scale= .982,
LKDNY7 No changes

34). EXITING LKDNY7- Modifications.
   Resources: WR= 0, RD= 0,
         CPU= 7.386, RTIME= 18.84,

35). ENTERING LKDNY8- Modifications
   1). EXITING LKDNY8. Results are: Conf= 1.000,
      Dx= 1.809, Dy= 1.328, Dz= -.067,
      Dist= 1.000, Scale= 1.068,
LKDNY8 Distance= .3590003. scale= 1.0245202

   2). EXITING LKDNY8. Results are: Conf= 1.000,
      Dx= .920, Dy= 1.097, Dz= -.174,
      Dist= -.895, Scale= .940,
LKDNY8 Distance= -.8947368. scale= .9403509

   3). EXITING LKDNY8. Results are: Conf= 1.000,
      Dx= 1.124, Dy= .536, Dz= -.247,
      Dist= -1.692, Scale= .880,
LKDNY8 No changes

35). EXITING LKDNY8- Modifications.
   Resources: WR= 0, RD= 0,
         CPU= 5.498, RTIME= 14.50,

36). ENTERING LKDNY9- Modifications
   1). EXITING LKDNY9. Results are: Conf= .857,
      Dx= 2.494, Dy= 1.769, Dz= -.140,
      Dist= -3.360, Scale= .491,
LKDNY9 Distance= -.6600000. scale= .9000000

   2). EXITING LKDNY9. Results are: Conf= .714,
      Dx= 2.490, Dy= 1.702, Dz= -.382,
      Dist= -1.200, Scale= .798,
LKDNY9 Distance= -.5940000. scale= .9000000

   3). EXITING LKDNY9. Results are: Conf= 1.000,
      Dx= -1.400, Dy= 1.014, Dz= -.395,
      Dist= -3.889, Scale= .273,
LKDNY9 No changes

36). EXITING LKDNY9- Modifications.
   Resources: WR= 0, RD= 0,
         CPU= 3.164, RTIME= 19.116,

37). ENTERING Left Kidney

   1). EXITING LKDNY1. Results are: Conf= .889,
      Dx= -.643, Dy= 1.298, Dz= .353,
      Dist= -2.703, Scale= .683,
   2). EXITING LKDNY2. Results are: Conf= 1.000,
      Dx= .325, Dy= .502, Dz= -.005,
      Dist= -1.225, Scale= .908,
   3). EXITING LKDNY3. Results are: Conf= 1.000,
      Dx= .387, Dy= .587, Dz= .001,
      Dist= -2.045, Scale= .891,
   4). EXITING LKDNY4. Results are: Conf= .789,
      Dx= -.203, Dy= .294, Dz= .007,
      Dist= -.167, Scale= .991,
   5). EXITING LKDNY5. Results are: Conf= .800,
      Dx= .222, Dy= -.162, Dz= -.041,
      Dist= -.182, Scale= .990,

6). EXITING LKDNY6. Results are: Conf= .789,
      Dx= .075, Dy= .192, Dz= -.035,
      Dist= -1.182, Scale= .935,
7). EXITING LKDNY7. Results are: Conf= 1.000,
      Dx= .600, Dy= .511, Dz= -.122,
      Dist= -.545, Scale= .968,
8). EXITING LKDNY8. Results are: Conf= 1.000,
      Dx= 1.561, Dy= .823, Dz= -.038,
      Dist= -1.154, Scale= .918,
9). EXITING LKDNY9. Results are: Conf= .833,
      Dx= -.743, Dy= 1.507, Dz= -.590,
      Dist= -2.127, Scale= .602,

10). EXITING Zscan of LKDNY1.
      Results are: Conf= .556, Zdisp= 1.625,
11). EXITING Zscan of LKDNY9.
      Results are: Conf= .833, Zdisp= -.111,

37). EXITING Left Kidney.
      Resources: WR= 0, RD= 228,
                 CPU= 20.914, RTIME= 1:20.166,
      Results are: Conf= .694, Dcnf= .000, Dx= .000,
      Dz= .000, Dy= .000, Scnf= .694,
      Sx= 1.000, Sy= 1.000, Sz= .978,
      = .006, = .003, = 1.000,

Org scale (1.0000000, 1.0000000, .9782986)
new size: (40.000000 40.000000 102.29171).

38). ENTERING Left Kidney
      1). EXITING LKDNY1. Results are: Conf= 1.000,
            Dx= .377, Dy= 2.477, Dz= .652,
            Dist= 1.167, Scale= 1.137,
      2). EXITING LKDNY2. Results are: Conf= 1.000,
            Dx= .377, Dy= .397, Dz= -.003,
            Dist= -1.140, Scale= .915,
      3). EXITING LKDNY3. Results are: Conf= 1.000,
            Dx= .383, Dy= .975, Dz= -.010,
            Dist= -2.000, Scale= .893,
      4). EXITING LKDNY4. Results are: Conf= .789,
            Dx= -.203, Dy= .294, Dz= .007,
            Dist= -.167, Scale= .991,
      5). EXITING LKDNY5. Results are: Conf= .800,
            Dx= .222, Dy= -.162, Dz= -.041,
            Dist= -.182, Scale= .990,
      6). EXITING LKDNY6. Results are: Conf= .789,
            Dx= .075, Dy= .342, Dz= -.045,
            Dist= -1.182, Scale= .935,
      7). EXITING LKDNY7. Results are: Conf= 1.000,
            Dx= .601, Dy= .558, Dz= -.124,
            Dist= -.415, Scale= .976,
      8). EXITING LKDNY8. Results are: Conf= 1.000,
            Dx= 1.309, Dy= .710, Dz= -.031,
            Dist= .077, Scale= 1.005,
      9). EXITING LKDNY9. Results are: Conf= 1.000,
            Dx= -.750, Dy= .614, Dz= -.321,
            Dist= -1.609, Scale= .699,

      10). EXITING Zscan of LKDNY1.
            Results are: Conf= .556, Zdisp= .625,
      11). EXITING Zscan of LKDNY9.
            Results are: Conf= .667, Zdisp= 1.000,

38). EXITING Left Kidney.
      Resources: WR= 0, RD= 21,
                 CPU= 18.874, RTIME= 1:0.900,
      Results are: Conf= .611, Dcnf= .611, Dx= .000,
      Dz= .813, Dy= .000, Scnf= .000,
      Sx= 1.000, Sy= 1.000, Sz= 1.000,
      = .000, = -.007, = 1.000,

Org disp(.0000000, .0000000, 1.0000000),
      new center is: (82.1723220,79.4665050,-59.2222220).

39). ENTERING Left Kidney
      1). EXITING LKDNY1. Results are: Conf= 1.000,
            Dx= -1.393, Dy= 1.954, Dz= .552,
            Dist= 2.833, Scale= 1.332,
      2). EXITING LKDNY2. Results are: Conf= 1.000,
            Dx= .377, Dy= .397, Dz= -.003,
            Dist= -1.140, Scale= .915,
      3). EXITING LKDNY3. Results are: Conf= 1.000,
            Dx= .005, Dy= .446, Dz= -.014,
            Dist= -1.105, Scale= .941,
      4). EXITING LKDNY4. Results are: Conf= .789,
            Dx= -.203, Dy= .294, Dz= .007,
            Dist= -.167, Scale= .991,
      5). EXITING LKDNY5. Results are: Conf= .800,
            Dx= .222, Dy= -.162, Dz= -.041,
            Dist= -.182, Scale= .990,
      6). EXITING LKDNY6. Results are: Conf= .789,
            Dx= .524, Dy= -.140, Dz= -.151,
            Dist= -1.462, Scale= .920,
      7). EXITING LKDNY7. Results are: Conf= 1.000,
            Dx= .712, Dy= .178, Dz= -.138,
            Dist= -.374, Scale= .978,
      8). EXITING LKDNY8. Results are: Conf= 1.000,
            Dx= 1.309, Dy= .710, Dz= -.031,
            Dist= .077, Scale= 1.005,
      9). EXITING LKDNY9. Results are: Conf= .833,
            Dx= -.741, Dy= 1.504, Dz= -.601,
            Dist= -2.127, Scale= .602,

      10). EXITING Zscan of LKDNY1.
            Results are: Conf= .667, Zdisp= -.500,
      11). EXITING Zscan of LKDNY9.
            Results are: Conf= .833, Zdisp= .333,

39). EXITING Left Kidney.
      Resources: WR= 0, RD= 138,
                 CPU= 21.661, RTIME= 1:18.950,
      Results are: Conf= .000, Dcnf= .000, Dx= .000,
      Dz= .000, Dy= .000, Scnf= .000,
      Sx= 1.000, Sy= 1.000, Sz= 1.000,
      Orientation= [.012,-.002, 1.000]

Organ - No changes

40). ENTERING LKDNY1- Modifications
      1). EXITING LKDNY1. Results are: Conf= 1.000,
            Dx= -1.393, Dy= 1.954, Dz= .552,
            Dist= 2.833, Scale= 1.332,
LKDNY1 Distance= .4763117. scale= 1.0558809

      2). EXITING LKDNY1. Results are: Conf= 1.000,
            Dx= -1.513, Dy= 2.736, Dz= .785,
            Dist= 3.200, Scale= 1.356,
LKDNY1 No changes

40). EXITING LKDNY1- Modifications.
      Resources: WR= 0, RD= 5,
                 CPU= 3.193, RTIME= 11.517,

41). ENTERING LKDNY2- Modifications
      1). EXITING LKDNY2. Results are: Conf= 1.000,
            Dx= .377, Dy= .397, Dz= -.003,
            Dist= -1.140, Scale= .915,
LKDNY2 Distance= -1.1404683. scale= .9147735

      2). EXITING LKDNY2. Results are: Conf= 1.000,
            Dx= .658, Dy= -.138, Dz= -.048,
            Dist= -.389, Scale= .968,

LKDNY2 disp= (.6576020,-.1379685)= .6719194
    New center= [3.1376356, .7673684].

    3). EXITING LKDNY2. Results are: Conf= 1.000,
        Dx= -.314, Dy= .153, Dz= .040,
        Dist= .512, Scale= 1.042,
LKDNY2 Distance= .5116280. scale= 1.0417958

    4). EXITING LKDNY2. Results are: Conf= 1.000,
        Dx= -.381, Dy= .197, Dz= .072,
        Dist= .846, Scale= 1.066,
LKDNY2 Distance= .8461539. scale= 1.0663506

    5). EXITING LKDNY2. Results are: Conf= 1.000,
        Dx= -.632, Dy= .051, Dz= .206,
        Dist= 1.000, Scale= 1.074,
LKDNY2 Distance= 1.0000001. scale= 1.0735352

    6). EXITING LKDNY2. Results are: Conf= 1.000,
        Dx= -1.063, Dy= .098, Dz= .443,
        Dist= 1.111, Scale= 1.076,
LKDNY2 No changes

    41). EXITING LKDNY2- Modifications.
        Resources: WR= 0, RD= 145,
                CPU= 13.7, RTIME= 1:1.684,

    42). ENTERING LKDNY3- Modifications
        1). EXITING LKDNY3. Results are: Conf= 1.000,
            Dx= .005, Dy= .446, Dz= -.014,
            Dist= -1.105, Scale= .941,
LKDNY3 Distance= -1.1052633. scale= .9410302

    2). EXITING LKDNY3. Results are: Conf= 1.000,
        Dx= -.031, Dy= -.331, Dz= .023,
        Dist= .067, Scale= 1.004,
LKDNY3 disp= (-.0308328,-.3314774)= .3329083
    New center= [1.3006451, 1.9762963].

    3). EXITING LKDNY3. Results are: Conf= 1.000,
        Dx= -.616, Dy= -.139, Dz= .081,
        Dist= .750, Scale= 1.043,
LKDNY3 Distance= .7499999. scale= 1.0425228

    4). EXITING LKDNY3. Results are: Conf= 1.000,
        Dx= -.373, Dy= .043, Dz= .065,
        Dist= .200, Scale= 1.011,
LKDNY3 No changes

    42). EXITING LKDNY3- Modifications.
        Resources: WR= 0, RD= 0,
                CPU= 7.477, RTIME= 18.466,

    43). ENTERING LKDNY4- Modifications
        1). EXITING LKDNY4. Results are: Conf= .789,
            Dx= -.203, Dy= .294, Dz= .007,
            Dist= -.167, Scale= .991,
LKDNY4 No changes

    43). EXITING LKDNY4- Modifications.
        Resources: WR= 0, RD= 0,
                CPU= 1.794, RTIME= 4.84,

    44). ENTERING LKDNY5- Modifications
        1). EXITING LKDNY5. Results are: Conf= .800,
            Dx= .222, Dy= -.162, Dz= -.041,
            Dist= -.182, Scale= .990,
LKDNY5 No changes

    44). EXITING LKDNY5- Modifications.
        Resources: WR= 0, RD= 0,
                CPU= 1.506, RTIME= 2.800,

    45). ENTERING LKDNY6- Modifications
        1). EXITING LKDNY6. Results are: Conf= .789,
            Dx= .524, Dy= -.140, Dz= -.151,
            Dist= -1.462, Scale= .920,
LKDNY6 Distance= -1.4615385. scale= .9200153

    2). EXITING LKDNY6. Results are: Conf= .778,
        Dx= .181, Dy= -.346, Dz= -.037,
        Dist= .333, Scale= 1.020,
LKDNY6 Distance= .3333334. scale= 1.0198281

    3). EXITING LKDNY6. Results are: Conf= .778,
        Dx= .227, Dy= -.258, Dz= -.076,
        Dist= -.053, Scale= .997,
LKDNY6 No changes

    45). EXITING LKDNY6- Modifications.
        Resources: WR= 0, RD= 0,
                CPU= 6.348, RTIME= 18.700,

    46). ENTERING LKDNY7- Modifications
        1). EXITING LKDNY7. Results are: Conf= 1.000,
            Dx= .712, Dy= .178, Dz= -.138,
            Dist= -.374, Scale= .978,
LKDNY7 Distance= -.3739130. scale= .9783766

    2). EXITING LKDNY7. Results are: Conf= 1.000,
        Dx= .660, Dy= .139, Dz= -.189,
        Dist= -.590, Scale= .965,
LKDNY7 Distance= -.5897437. scale= .9651413

    3). EXITING LKDNY7. Results are: Conf= 1.000,
        Dx= .996, Dy= -.176, Dz= -.346,
        Dist= 1.091, Scale= 1.067,
LKDNY7 Distance= 1.0909091. scale= 1.0668106

    4). EXITING LKDNY7. Results are: Conf= 1.000,
        Dx= .273, Dy= .930, Dz= -.250,
        Dist= -.121, Scale= .993,
LKDNY7 No changes

    46). EXITING LKDNY7- Modifications.
        Resources: WR= 0, RD= 0,
                CPU= 7.766, RTIME= 24.500,

    47). ENTERING LKDNY8- Modifications
        1). EXITING LKDNY8. Results are: Conf= 1.000,
            Dx= 1.309, Dy= .710, Dz= -.031,
            Dist= .077, Scale= 1.005,
LKDNY8 No changes

    47). EXITING LKDNY8- Modifications.
        Resources: WR= 0, RD= 0,
                CPU= 1.673, RTIME= 4.517,

    48). ENTERING LKDNY9- Modifications
        1). EXITING LKDNY9. Results are: Conf= .833,
            Dx= -.741, Dy= 1.504, Dz= -.601,
            Dist= -2.127, Scale= .602,
LKDNY9 Distance= -.5346000. scale= .9000000

    2). EXITING LKDNY9. Results are: Conf= .833,
        Dx= 1.093, Dy= .378, Dz= -.036,
        Dist= -2.000, Scale= .584,
LKDNY9 Distance= -.3113999. scale= .9352787

    3). EXITING LKDNY9. Results are: Conf= .833,
        Dx= 1.268, Dy= .880, Dz= -.334,
        Dist= -2.623, Scale= .417,
LKDNY9 disp= (.2576093, .2576093)= .3643146
    New center= [3.6832333, 2.4795274].

4). EXITING LKDNY9. **Results are:** Conf= .833,
　　　　Dx= 1.235, Dy= .866, Dz= -.467,
　　　　Dist= -2.623, Scale= .417,
LKDNY9 disp= (.2576093, .2576093)= .3643146
New center= [3.9408426, 2.7371368].

5). **EXITING LKDNY9. Results are:** Conf= 1.000,
　　　　Dx= -.038, Dy= .363, Dz= -.169,
　　　　Dist= -1.587, Scale= .647,

LKDNY9 No changes

48). EXITING LKDNY9- Modifications.
　　　　Resources: WR= 0, RD= 0,
　　　　　　　CPU= 3.802, RTIME= 27.717,

49). ENTERING Left Kidney
　　1). EXITING LKDNY1. Results are: Conf= 1.000,
　　　　Dx= -1.194, Dy= 1.131, Dz= .477,
　　　　Dist= 1.667, Scale= 1.185,
　　2). EXITING LKDNY2. Results are: Conf= 1.000,
　　　　Dx= -.294, Dy= 1.077, Dz= .011,
　　　　Dist= -2.000, Scale= .863,
　　3). EXITING LKDNY3. Results are: Conf= 1.000,
　　　　Dx= -.177, Dy= .306, Dz= -.025,
　　　　Dist= -.686, Scale= .963,
　　4). EXITING LKDNY4. Results are: Conf= .789,
　　　　Dx= -.090, Dy= .254, Dz= .002,
　　　　Dist= -.040, Scale= .998,
　　5). EXITING LKDNY5. Results are: Conf= .800,
　　　　Dx= .329, Dy= -.386, Dz= -.056,
　　　　Dist= -.238, Scale= .987,
　　6). EXITING LKDNY6. Results are: Conf= .778,
　　　　Dx= .479, Dy= -.438, Dz= -.118,
　　　　Dist= -.143, Scale= .992,
　　7). EXITING LKDNY7. Results are: Conf= 1.000,
　　　　Dx= .650, Dy= .208, Dz= -.127,
　　　　Dist= -.250, Scale= .986,
　　8). EXITING LKDNY8. Results are: Conf= 1.000,
　　　　Dx= 2.452, Dy= .553, Dz= -.091,
　　　　Dist= -.500, Scale= .965,
　　9). EXITING LKDNY9. Results are: Conf= .833,
　　　　Dx= .244, Dy= .391, Dz= -.134,
　　　　Dist= -.085, Scale= .981,

　10). EXITING Zscan of LKDNY1.
　　　　Results are: Conf= .600, Zdisp= -.364,
　11). EXITING Zscan of LKDNY9.
　　　　Results are: Conf= .800, Zdisp= .714,

49). EXITING Left Kidney.
　　　　Resources: WR= 0, RD= 249,
　　　　　　　CPU= 23.939, RTIME= 1:35.0,
　　　　Results are: Conf= .700, Dcnf= .000, Dx= .000,
　　　　Dz= .000, Dy= .000, Scnf= .700,
　　　　Sx= 1.000, Sy= 1.000, Sz= 1.013,
　　　　Orientation= [.024,-.008, 1.000]

Org scale (1.0000000, 1.0000000, 1.0134740)
new size: (40.000000 40.000000 103.66999).

50). ENTERING Left Kidney
　　1). EXITING LKDNY1. Results are: Conf= 1.000,
　　　　Dx= -.352, Dy= 2.496, Dz= .757,
　　　　Dist= -.667, Scale= .926,
　　2). EXITING LKDNY2. Results are: Conf= 1.000,
　　　　Dx= -.294, Dy= 1.077, Dz= .011,
　　　　Dist= -2.000, Scale= .863,
　　3). EXITING LKDNY3. Results are: Conf= 1.000,
　　　　Dx= -.088, Dy= .357, Dz= -.020,
　　　　Dist= -.914, Scale= .950,

4). EXITING LKDNY4. Results are: Conf= .789,
　　　　Dx= -.090, Dy= .254, Dz= .002,
　　　　Dist= -.040, Scale= .998,
5). EXITING LKDNY5. Results are: Conf= .800,
　　　　Dx= .329, Dy= -.386, Dz= -.055,
　　　　Dist= -.238, Scale= .987,
6). EXITING LKDNY6. Results are: Conf= .778,
　　　　Dx= .479, Dy= -.439, Dz= -.117,
　　　　Dist= -.143, Scale= .992,
7). EXITING LKDNY7. Results are: Conf= 1.000,
　　　　Dx= .484, Dy= .107, Dz= -.093,
　　　　Dist= -.526, Scale= .970,
8). EXITING LKDNY8. Results are: Conf= 1.000,
　　　　Dx= 2.491, Dy= .553, Dz= -.093,
　　　　Dist= -1.263, Scale= .910,
9). EXITING LKDNY9. Results are: Conf= .833,
　　　　Dx= 1.858, Dy= .545, Dz= -.051,
　　　　Dist= -1.712, Scale= .620,

10). EXITING Zscan of LKDNY1.
　　　　Results are: Conf= .700, Zdisp= -.545,
11). EXITING Zscan of LKDNY9.
　　　　Results are: Conf= .600, Zdisp= -1.400,

50). EXITING Left Kidney.
　　　　Resources: WR= 0, RD= 474,
　　　　　　　CPU= 29.984, RTIME= 2:5.850,
　　　　Results are: Conf= .650, Dcnf= .650, Dx= .0(
　　　　Dz= -.973, Dy= .000, Scnf= .000,
　　　　Sx= 1.000, Sy= 1.000, Sz= 1.000,
　　　　Orientation= [.026, -.014, 1.000]

Org disp(.0000000, .0000000,-1.0000000),
　　new center i:(21220 79.4665050,-60.2222220).

51). ENTERING Left Kidney
　　1). EXITING LKDNY1. Results are: Conf= 1.000,
　　　　Dx= -1.117, Dy= 1.791, Dz= .651,
　　　　Dist= -1.000, Scale= .889,
　　2). EXITING LKDNY2. Results are: Conf= 1.000,
　　　　Dx= -.294, Dy= 1.077, Dz= .011,
　　　　Dist= -2.000, Scale= .863,
　　3). EXITING LKDNY3. Results are: Conf= 1.000,
　　　　Dx= -.206, Dy= .569, Dz= -.037,
　　　　Dist= -1.111, Scale= .940,
　　4). EXITING LKDNY4. Results are: Conf= .789,
　　　　Dx= -.090, Dy= .254, Dz= .002,
　　　　Dist= -.040, Scale= .998,
　　5). EXITING LKDNY5. Results are: Conf= .800,
　　　　Dx= .329, Dy= -.386, Dz= -.055,
　　　　Dist= -.238, Scale= .987,
　　6). EXITING LKDNY6. Results are: Conf= .778,
　　　　Dx= .441, Dy= -.344, Dz= -.111,
　　　　Dist= .533, Scale= 1.031,
　　7). EXITING LKDNY7. Results are: Conf= 1.000,
　　　　Dx= .480, Dy= .271, Dz= -.095,
　　　　Dist= -.250, Scale= .986,
　　8). EXITING LKDNY8. Results are: Conf= 1.000,
　　　　Dx= 2.491, Dy= .553, Dz= -.093,
　　　　Dist= -1.263, Scale= .910,
　　9). EXITING LKDNY9. Results are: Conf= 1.000,
　　　　Dx= .001, Dy= .476, Dz= -.188,
　　　　Dist= -.356, Scale= .921,

　10). EXITING Zscan of LKDNY1.
　　　　Results are: Conf= .900, Zdisp= .923,
　11). EXITING Zscan of LKDNY9.
　　　　Results are: Conf= .800, Zdisp= .714,

51). EXITING Left Kidney.
　　　　Resources: WR= 0, RD= 168,
　　　　　　　CPU= 23.228, RTIME= 1:28.0,

Results are: Conf= .850, Dcnf= .850, Dx= .000,
   Dz= .819, Dy= .000, Scnf= .000,
   Sx= 1.000, Sy= 1.000, Sz= 1.000,
   Orientation= [.022, -.011, 1.000]

Org disp(.0000000, .0000000, 1.0000000),
   new center is:(21220 79.4665050,-59.2222220).

52). ENTERING Left Kidney
   1). EXITING LKDNY1. Results are: Conf= 1.000,
      Dx= -.352, Dy= 2.496, Dz= .757,
      Dist= -.667, Scale= .926,
   2). EXITING LKDNY2. Results are: Conf= 1.000,
      Dx= -.294, Dy= 1.077, Dz= .011,
      Dist= -2.000, Scale= .863,
   3). EXITING LKDNY3. Results are: Conf= 1.000,
      Dx= -.088, Dy= .357, Dz= -.020,
      Dist= -.914, Scale= .950,
   4). EXITING LKDNY4. Results are: Conf= .789,
      Dx= -.090, Dy= .254, Dz= .002,
      Dist= -.040, Scale= .998,
   5). EXITING LKDNY5. Results are: Conf= .800,

      Dx= .329, Dy= -.386, Dz= -.055,
      Dist= -.238, Scale= .987,
   6). EXITING LKDNY6. Results are: Conf= .778,
      Dx= .479, Dy= -.439, Dz= -.117,
      Dist= -.143, Scale= .992,
   7). EXITING LKDNY7. Results are: Conf= 1.000,
      Dx= .484, Dy= .107, Dz= -.093,
      Dist= -.526, Scale= .970,
   8). EXITING LKDNY8. Results are: Conf= 1.000,
      Dx= 2.491, Dy= .553, Dz= -.093,
      Dist= -1.263, Scale= .910,
   9). EXITING LKDNY9. Results are: Conf= .833,
      Dx= 1.858, Dy= .545, Dz= -.051,
      Dist= -1.712, Scale= .620,

   10). EXITING Zscan of LKDNY1.
      Results are: Conf= .700, Zdisp= -.545,
   11). EXITING Zscan of LKDNY9.
      Results are: Conf= .600, Zdisp= -1.400,

52). EXITING Left Kidney.
   Resources: WR= 0, RD= 180,
      CPU= 23.804, RTIME= 1:26.566,
   Results are: Conf= .650, Dcnf= .650, Dx= .0(
   Dz= -.973, Dy= .000, Scnf= .000,
   Sx= 1.000, Sy= 1.000, Sz= 1.000,
   Orientation= [.026, -.014, 1.000]

Organ oriented by [.0260327,-.0136197, .9995683].

53). ENTERING Left Kidney
   1). EXITING LKDNY1. Results are: Conf= 1.000,
      Dx= 1.077, Dy= .884, Dz= .104,
      Dist= -.125, Scale= .986,
   2). EXITING LKDNY2. Results are: Conf= 1.000,
      Dx= -.881, Dy= 1.224, Dz= .052,
      Dist= .071, Scale= 1.005,
   3). EXITING LKDNY3. Results are: Conf= 1.000,
      Dx= .204, Dy= .085, Dz= .008,
      Dist= -.056, Scale= .997,
   4). EXITING LKDNY4. Results are: Conf= .789,
      Dx= .024, Dy= -.055, Dz= -.002,
      Dist= -.040, Scale= .998,
   5). EXITING LKDNY5. Results are: Conf= .800,
      Dx= .133, Dy= .171, Dz= -.036,
      Dist= .556, Scale= 1.030,
   6). EXITING LKDNY6. Results are: Conf= .778,
      Dx= .118, Dy= -.389, Dz= -.020,
      Dist= .500, Scale= 1.029,

7). EXITING LKDNY7. Results are: Conf= 1.000,
   Dx= .662, Dy= .845, Dz= -.147,
   Dist= -1.053, Scale= .940,
8). EXITING LKDNY8. Results are: Conf= 1.000,
   Dx= .742, Dy= .958, Dz= -.104,
   Dist= -.526, Scale= .963,
9). EXITING LKDNY9. Results are: Conf= 1.000,
   Dx= .924, Dy= -.062, Dz= .080,
   Dist= 1.455, Scale= 1.323,

10). EXITING Zscan of LKDNY1.
   Results are: Conf= .900, Zdisp= -.700,
11). EXITING Zscan of LKDNY9.
   Results are: Conf= .600, Zdisp= -1.200,

53). EXITING Left Kidney.
   Resources: WR= 0, RD= 282,
      CPU= 26.684, RTIME= 1:45.416,
   Results are: Conf= .750, Dcnf= .750, Dx= .000,
   Dz= -.950, Dy= .000, Scnf= .000,
   Sx= 1.000, Sy= 1.000, Sz= 1.000,
   Orientation= [.009, -.004, 1.000]

Organ - No changes

54). ENTERING LKDNY1- Modifications
   1). EXITING LKDNY1. Results are: Conf= 1.000,
      Dx= 1.077, Dy= .884, Dz= .104,
      Dist= -.125, Scale= .986,
LKDNY1 disp= (1.0766419, .8842639)= 1.3932267
   New center= [3.9316956, 3.7427920].

   2). EXITING LKDNY1. Results are: Conf= 1.000,
      Dx= -1.953, Dy= 1.260, Dz= .869,
      Dist= -.681, Scale= .924,
LKDNY1 disp= (-.5125978, 1.0777617)= 1.1934517
   New center= [3.4190977, 4.8205537].

   3). EXITING LKDNY1. Results are: Conf= 1.000,
      Dx= .188, Dy= 1.058, Dz= .214,
      Dist= -1.727, Scale= .808,
LKDNY1 disp= (.1884185, 1.0584560)= 1.0750956
   New center= [3.6075162, 5.8790097].

   4). EXITING LKDNY1. Results are: Conf= 1.000,
      Dx= -.048, Dy= -.615, Dz= -.135,
      Dist= -2.610, Scale= .710,
LKDNY1 No changes

54). EXITING LKDNY1- Modifications.
   Resources: WR= 0, RD= 4,
      CPU= 4.823, RTIME= 25.384,

55). ENTERING LKDNY2- Modifications
   1). EXITING LKDNY2. Results are: Conf= 1.000,
      Dx= -.881, Dy= 1.224, Dz= .052,
      Dist= .071, Scale= 1.005,
LKDNY2 disp= (-.8810097, .5119742)= 1.0189544
   New center= [2.2566259, 1.2793156].

   2). EXITING LKDNY2. Results are: Conf= 1.000,
      Dx= -.655, Dy= .739, Dz= .089,
      Dist= -1.000, Scale= .932,
LKDNY2 disp= (-.6554763, .5119742)= .8317085
   New center= [1.6011496, 1.7912627].

   3). EXITING LKDNY2. Results are: Conf= 1.000,
      Dx= -.010, Dy= .502, Dz= -.008,
      Dist= -.647, Scale= .956,
LKDNY2 disp= (.0000000, .5021384)= .5021384
   New center= [1.6011496, 2.2934011].

4). EXITING LKDNY2. Results are: Conf= 1.000,
    Dx= .003, Dy= -.551, Dz= .023,
    Dist= .333, Scale= 1.023,
LKDNY2 Distance= .3333335. scale= 1.0228327

5). EXITING LKDNY2. Results are: Conf= 1.000,
    Dx= -.124, Dy= -.401, Dz= .089,
    Dist= .512, Scale= 1.034,
LKDNY2 Distance= .0677392. scale= 1.0045364

6). EXITING LKDNY2. Results are: Conf= 1.000,
    Dx= -.803, Dy= -1.167, Dz= .620,
    Dist= -.305, Scale= .980,
LKDNY2 No changes

55). EXITING LKDNY2- Modifications.
    Resources: WR= 1, RD= 462,
        CPU= 27.913, RTIME= 2:13.200,

56). ENTERING LKDNY3- Modifications
    1). EXITING LKDNY3. Results are: Conf= 1.000,
    Dx= .204, Dy= .085, Dz= .008,
    Dist= -.056, Scale= .997,
LKDNY3 No changes

56). EXITING LKDNY3- Modifications.
    Resources: WR= 0, RD= 77,
        CPU= 4.622, RTIME= 21.684,

57). ENTERING LKDNY4- Modifications
    1). EXITING LKDNY4. Results are: Conf= .789,
    Dx= .024, Dy= -.055, Dz= -.002,
    Dist= -.040, Scale= .998,
LKDNY4 No changes

57). EXITING LKDNY4- Modifications.
    Resources: WR= 0, RD= 9, CPU= 1.738, RTIME= 3.783,

58). ENTERING LKDNY5- Modifications
    1). EXITING LKDNY5. Results are: Conf= .800,
    Dx= .133, Dy= .171, Dz= -.036,
    Dist= .556, Scale= 1.030,
LKDNY5 Distance= .5555555. scale= 1.0295433

2). EXITING LKDNY5. Results are: Conf= .800,
    Dx= .206, Dy= .118, Dz= -.078,
    Dist= -1.000, Scale= .948,
LKDNY5 Distance= -1.0000000. scale= .9483480

3). EXITING LKDNY5. Results are: Conf= .789,
    Dx= .138, Dy= -.083, Dz= -.060,
    Dist= .400, Scale= 1.022,
LKDNY5 Distance= .4000001. scale= 1.0217861

4). EXITING LKDNY5. Results are: Conf= .789,
    Dx= .110, Dy= -.329, Dz= -.036,
    Dist= .167, Scale= 1.009,
LKDNY5 No changes

58). EXITING LKDNY5- Modifications.
    Resources: WR= 0, RD= 46,
        CPU= 10.417, RTIME= 38.417,

59). ENTERING LKDNY6- Modifications
    1). EXITING LKDNY6. Results are: Conf= .778,
    Dx= .118, Dy= -.389, Dz= -.020,
    Dist= .500, Scale= 1.029,
LKDNY6 Distance= .5000001. scale= 1.0291638

2). EXITING LKDNY6. Results are: Conf= .778,
    Dx= .080, Dy= -.411, Dz= -.005,
    Dist= -.111, Scale= .994,
LKDNY6 No changes

59). EXITING LKDNY6- Modifications.
    Resources: WR= 0, RD= 0,
        CPU= 5.406, RTIME= 18.767,

60). ENTERING LKDNY7- Modifications
    1). EXITING LKDNY7. Results are: Conf= 1.000,
    Dx= .662, Dy= .845, Dz= -.147,
    Dist= -1.053, Scale= .940,
LKDNY7 Distance= -1.0526316. scale= .9395709

2). EXITING LKDNY7. Results are: Conf= 1.000,
    Dx= .753, Dy= -.063, Dz= -.246,
    Dist= -.062, Scale= .996,
LKDNY7 No changes

60). EXITING LKDNY7- Modifications.
    Resources: WR= 0, RD= 0,
        CPU= 4.869, RTIME= 17.800,

61). ENTERING LKDNY8- Modifications
    1). EXITING LKDNY8. Results are: Conf= 1.000,
    Dx= .742, Dy= .958, Dz= -.104,
    Dist= -.526, Scale= .963,
LKDNY8 Distance= -.5263158. scale= .9626866

2). EXITING LKDNY8. Results are: Conf= 1.000,
    Dx= .260, Dy= .649, Dz= -.103,
    Dist= -.750, Scale= .945,
LKDNY8 Distance= -.7500000. scale= .9447675

3). EXITING LKDNY8. Results are: Conf= 1.000,
    Dx= -.089, Dy= .287, Dz= -.012,
    Dist= -.333, Scale= .974,
LKDNY8 No changes

61). EXITING LKDNY8- Modifications.
    Resources: WR= 0, RD= 0,
        CPU= 5.981, RTIME= 18.383,

62). ENTERING LKDNY9- Modifications
    1). EXITING LKDNY9. Results are: Conf= 1.00(
    Dx= .924, Dy= -.062, Dz= .080,
    Dist= 1.455, Scale= 1.323,
LKDNY9 Distance= .4500000. scale= 1.1000000

2). EXITING LKDNY9. Results are: Conf= .833,
    Dx= .565, Dy= .312, Dz= -.151,
    Dist= -.873, Scale= .824,
LKDNY9 Distance= -.4500000. scale= .9090909

3). EXITING LKDNY9. Results are: Conf= 1.000,
    Dx= .051, Dy= -.120, Dz= .044,
    Dist= 1.807, Scale= 1.402,
LKDNY9 Distance= .4500000. scale= 1.1000000

4). EXITING LKDNY9. Results are: Conf= 1.000,
    Dx= -.342, Dy= -.329, Dz= .246,
    Dist= -1.127, Scale= .772,
LKDNY9 No changes

62). EXITING LKDNY9- Modifications.
    Resources: WR= 0, RD= 0,
        CPU= 3.597, RTIME= 19.733,

Exhaust major organ iterations

Listing E.3: Modifications trace of left kidney fit

```
Listing E.3:  Modifications-trace of lft kidney fit
0). No organ change
1). Organ Scale by [ 1.0000000,  1.0000000,  1.1000000].
2). Organ Scale by [ 1.0000000,  1.0000000,  1.1000000].
3). Organ Scale by [ 1.0000000,  1.0000000,  1.0847107].
4). No organ change
5). Organ displacement by [ 1.6677151,  3.1144838, -7.5000000].
6). Organ Oriented in direction: [ .0194645, .0054905, .9997955].
7). Organ Oriented in direction: [ .0174303, .0099584, .9997985].
8). No organ change
9). Slice1 displaced by [ .8855479, -1.0766602].
10). Slice1 displaced by [ 1.0766602, -1.0766602].
11). Slice1 Scaled by [ 1.1000000,  1.1000000].
12). Slice1 Scaled by [ 1.1000000,  1.1000000].
13). Slice1 Scaled by [ 1.1000000,  1.1000000].
14). Slice1 -- nothing
15). Slice2 displaced by [ 1.0766602, -.2366234].
16). Slice2 displaced by [ .5923643,  1.0766602].
17). Slice2 displaced by [ .5205105,  .6221542].
18). Slice2 Scaled by [ 1.1000000,  1.1000000].
19). Slice2 Scaled by [ 1.1000000,  1.1000000].
20). Slice2 displaced by [ .8681853,  .0000000].
21). Slice2 Scaled by [ 1.1000000,  1.1000000].
22). Slice2 displaced by [ 1.0766602,  .0000000].
23). Slice2 Scaled by [ 1.1000000,  1.1000000].
24). Slice2 Scaled by [ 1.0245202,  1.0245202].
25). Slice2 -- nothing
26). Slice3 displaced by [ .7648524,  .5221290].
27). Slice3 displaced by [ .3961484,  .0625581].
28). Slice3 -- nothing
29). Slice4 Scaled by [ .9000000,  .9000000].
30). Slice4 Scaled by [ .9000000,  .9000000].
31). Slice4 displaced by [ .3907083,  .8807178].
32). Slice4 displaced by [ .1421422,  .3846060].
33). Slice4 -- nothing
34). Slice5 Scaled by [ .9000000,  .9000000].
35). Slice5 displaced by [ .2338089,  2.0000000].
36). Slice5 displaced by [ .7801837,  1.5613566].
37). Slice5 displaced by [ 1.0127017,  1.3064040].
38). Slice5 -- nothing
39). Slice6 Scaled by [ .9000000,  .9000000].
40). Slice6 displaced by [ .7228338, -.1036658].
41). Slice6 -- nothing
42). Slice7 Scaled by [ 1.1000000,  1.1000000].
43). Slice7 displaced by [-.0328563, -.3689706].
44). Slice7 Scaled by [ 1.0395257,  1.0395257].
45). Slice7 Scaled by [ 1.0526334,  1.0526334].
46). Slice7 -- nothing
47). Slice8 Scaled by [ 1.1000000,  1.1000000].
48). Slice8 Scaled by [ 1.1000000,  1.1000000].
49). Slice8 Scaled by [ 1.1000000,  1.1000000].
50). Slice8 Scaled by [ 1.1000000,  1.1000000].
51). Slice8 Scaled by [ 1.0245202,  1.0245202].
52). Slice8 -- nothing
53). Slice9 Scaled by [ 1.1000000,  1.1000000].
54). Slice9 displaced by [ 1.0061194,  1.0766602].
55). Slice9 Scaled by [ 1.1000000,  1.1000000].
56). Slice9 displaced by [ .7332479,  1.0766602].
57). Slice9 Scaled by [ 1.1000000,  1.1000000].
58). Slice9 displaced by [ .0000000,  1.0766602].
59). Slice9 Scaled by [ 1.1000000,  1.1000000].
60). Slice9 displaced by [ .0000000,  .3826522].
61). Slice9 Scaled by [ 1.0245202,  1.0245202].
62). Slice9 -- nothing
63). Organ Oriented in direction: [-.0182243,-.0043171, .9998246].
64). No organ change
65). Slice1 Scaled by [ .9463347,  .9463347].
66). Slice1 Scaled by [ 1.1000000,  1.1000000].
```

```
 67). Slice1 -- nothing
 68). Slice2 -- nothing
 69). Slice3 -- nothing
 70). Slice4 -- nothing
 71). Slice5 Scaled by [ .9000000,   .9000000].
 72). Slice5 Scaled by [ 1.0326605,  1.0326605].
 73). Slice5 displaced by [ .6628012,   .2866367].
 74). Slice5 -- nothing
 75). Slice6 Scaled by [ .9000000,   .9000000].
 76). Slice6 displaced by [ 1.0282634,   .3797395].
 77). Slice6 -- nothing
 78). Slice7 displaced by [-.2494776,   .4480377].
 79). Slice7 Scaled by [ .9610564,   .9610564].
 80). Slice7 -- nothing
 81). Slice8 -- nothing
 82). Slice9 -- nothing
 83). No organ change
 84). Slice1 Scaled by [ .9000000,   .9000000].
 85). Slice1 Scaled by [ 1.1000000,  1.1000000].
 86). Slice1 -- nothing
 87). Slice2 -- nothing
 88). Slice3 -- nothing
 89). Slice4 -- nothing
 90). Slice5 -- nothing
 91). Slice6 -- nothing
 92). Slice7 -- nothing
 93). Slice8 -- nothing
 94). Slice9 -- nothing
 95). No organ change
 96). Slice1 Scaled by [ .9000000,   .9000000].
 97). Slice1 Scaled by [ 1.1000000,  1.1000000].
 98). Slice1 -- nothing
 99). Slice2 -- nothing
100). Slice3 -- nothing
101). Slice4 -- nothing
102). Slice5 -- nothing
103). Slice6 -- nothing
104). Slice7 -- nothing
105). Slice8 -- nothing
106). Slice9 -- nothing
107). No organ change
```

Appendix F

Generalized-Cylinders Manipulations

F.1 Introduction

Appendix F provides complementary technical details for the mathematical foundation of GC's as used in this study. These foundations include, first, a solution to the geometric transformation of a cross-section curve in the definition of a GC; and, second, a constraint formula that will keep a modified GC which is initially correct consistent with the definition of GC's (II.3.3) and eliminate potential pathological cases such as those in Figure 2.8A.

F.2 Cross-Sectional Transformation

Section II.3.1 presented the GC theory according to Agin. In Agin's solution, the orientation of a cross section is specified by two orthogonal vectors, $\vec{X}$ and $\vec{Y}$, that define a space-oriented coordinate system for the 2-D definition of a cross-section curve as it is "swept" along the main axis. These two axis vectors are perpendicular to a third vector, $\vec{Z}$, which is the tangent to the main axis curve of the GC. These vectors are the solution of a set of differential equations (Fernet Equations) based on the torsion and curvature of the analytic definition of the main axis curve and some initial conditions for the three vectors at the starting end of the main axis.

   In our case, because the main axis is a piece-wise polynomial, Agin's approach can be applied to each piece separately. Since the endpoint of one piece is the starting point of the next one, a solution at the end-point of one piece provides the initial condition for the next piece. Each piece is a parametric uniform cubic polynomial, and a uniform solution that depends only on a few parameters is achievable for all cases. The main problem with this approach is that Eq. 2.4 may be ill conditioned.

   To surmount this difficulty, we take a different approach, which provides an efficient and satisfactory solution. In this method, an affine transformation from the initial orientation (that of the cross-sectional curve at the beginning of a piece) to the one at its other end is calculated. Referring back to Eq. 2.4, only Θ degrees of in-plane rotation is allowed while the cross section is swept. If $\Theta =$

0, then such a rotation should be eliminated by designing the affine transformation in an appropriate way. As explained earlier, these transformations are defined piecewise, one for every endpoint of a main axis curve segment, relative to the given initial transformation at the beginning of the segment. To calculate the orientation of a particular cross section, we concatenate the relative orientations of all appropriate consecutive cross sections, beginning with the orientation for the first one. To complete the definition of a transformation for a planar cross-section curve to its position in the 3-D space of a GC, its orientation is concatenated with a translation of its centroid point [0,0,0] to the location of the appropriate knot point on the main axis curve, $\vec{A}(s)$. Transformations are defined as 4×4 matrixes, and concatenations performed by matrix multiplications [Newman, 1979]. The orientation problem is divided into two simpler problems:

1. The basic orientation problem and

2. The inter-cross-section problem.

F.2.1 The basic orientation problem

Problem F.1:

> Given a planar curve that is defined on the X-Y plane of a right-hand Cartesian coordinate system, and a vector, $\vec{A}$, find a transformation, T, that will orient the curve's plane so that it will be perpendicular to the vector $\vec{A}$. The transformation must not include in-plane rotations.

In general, a solution to this problem is a function that takes a vector parameter $\vec{A}$ and returns the matrix T: $T =$ Basic Orientation $(\vec{A})$.

Solution F1: In other words, the problem is to orient a unit vector $\vec{k}$ (in the $\vec{Z}$ direction) to the direction of $\vec{A}$. Thus, the X-Y plane to which $\vec{k}$ is normal, will be oriented perpendicularly to $\vec{A}$. We define a rotational transformation T which rotates around vector $\vec{V}$ by angle α where

$$\vec{V} = \vec{k} \times \vec{A'}$$
$$\alpha = \arccos (\vec{k} \cdot \vec{A'}) \qquad \text{(F.1A)}$$
$$\vec{A'} = \vec{A} / |A|$$

If $\vec{A'} = [a\ b\ c\ 1]$, then $\vec{V} = [0\ 0\ 1\ 1] \times [a\ b\ c\ 1] = [-b\ a\ 0\ 1]$

We define

$$CS = \cos (\alpha) \qquad \text{(F.1B)}$$
$$Sn = \sin (\alpha)$$

So the transformation is [Newman, 1979]:

$$T = \begin{bmatrix} b^2 + Cs \cdot (1 - b^2) & -a.b.(1-Cs) & a.Sn & 0 \\ -a.b.(1-Cs) & a^2 + Cs.(1-a^2) & b.Sn & 0 \\ -a.Sn & -b.Sn & Cs & 0 \\ 0 & 0 & 0 & 1 \end{bmatrix} \qquad (F.1C)$$

F.2.2 The Inter-cross-sectional Orientation Problem

Problem F.2:

Given two consecutive cross sections in the GC: C_1 and C_2. C_1 is oriented by a transformation $Trans_{C_1}$ to be perpendicular to the vector $\vec{N}_1$. C_2 is desired to be oriented perpendicular to the vector $\vec{N}_2$ ($\vec{N}_1$ and $\vec{N}_2$ are tangents to the main axis curve of the GC in the center points of the corresponding cross sections). Find a transformation that will orient C_1 from a position perpendicular to $\vec{N}_1$ to a position perpendicular to $\vec{N}_2$. This orientation must not introduce in-plane rotations.

Solution F.2:

This transformation is done in three steps:

1. Transform the coordinate system so that its Z axis will be parallel to $\vec{N}_1$.

2. In the new coordinate system, solve the basic orientation problem: orient the X-Y plane to be perpendicular to the new $\vec{N}_2$.

3. Invert the transformation done in (1).

The transformation in (1) is the inverse of the solution to the basic orientation problem for $\vec{N}_1$, called $Trans_{N_1}$. Its effect is equivalent (according to the theorem) to performing $Trans_{N_1}^{-1}$ on $\vec{N}_2$. Thus, the transformation in (3) is equivalent to performing $Trans_{N_1}$.

Therefore, the algorithm will be:

1. $Trans_{N_1} :=$ Basic Orientation (N_1);
   new $N_2 := Trans_{N_1}^{-1}(N_2)$;

2. $Trans_{N_{1,2}} :=$ Basic Orientation (*new* N_2);

3. $Trans_{C_{1,2}} :=$ Concatenate ($Trans_{N_1}^{-1}$, $Trans_{N_{1,2}}$, $Trans_{N_1}$).

where T^{-1} is the inverse transformation of T.

Finally, the orientation of C_2 will be the concatenation of the orientation for C_1 and the inter-cross-sectional orientation:

$$Trans_{C_2} := Concatenate\ (Trans_{C_1},\ Trans_{C_{1,2}}).$$

In the context of problem F.2, for the orientation of the first cross section of the GC (where s, the main axis parameter, is 0), $Trans_{C_1}$ is the trivial identity transformation I, and $\vec{N}_1$ is the Z axis. In practice, since each transformation is represented by a 4×4 matrix, all the orientations for the individual cross sections of a GC are calculated in one step by a routine call and returned as a list of matrices, one for each cross section. Note that no displacements are involved in these transformations. The reason is that, to calculate normals to the GC surface, only the cross-section orientation alone is needed, while in order to find locations on that surface, the displacement transformation is concatenated with the orientation.

Given a GC, algorithm F.1 provides the orientations. It is written in pidgin SAIL [Reiser, 1976]. The procedure *GCorient* takes a list parameter, *GC*, and returns a list of orientations.

Algorithm F.1

```
list procedure GCorient(list GC);
  begin
  list Orientations;
  real array Trans, Trans1, N1, N2 [1:4, 1:4];

  Orientations:= PHI;  COMMENT the empty list;
  Trans := I; COMMENT the identity transformation;
  N1 := [0,0,1]; COMMENT vector in the Z direction;

  for each Cross Section in GC do
     begin
     N2 := Normal!Of (Cross Section);
     Trans 1 := Inter!CS!orientation (N1, N2);
     Trans := Concatenate (Trans, Trans1);

     put Trans in Orientations;

     N1 := N2;
     end;
  end;
```

F.3 Curvature Constraints on GC's

The basic approach to 3-D image analysis as taken here is to iteratively match and modify a GC, starting with a correct, syntactic one. In this section we shall be concerned with the prevention of pathological cases as in Figure 2.8A. For this purpose we consider a restricted case of a GC, called "discrete GC," in which this consistency is assured only at knot points of the main axis curve. At each knot point of the main axis curve, the radius of the corresponding cross section must be smaller than the radius of curvature (ρ) of the main axis curve. If this condition is checked at every knot point, our intuition is that it will ensure correctness all along the main axis curve. Since we don't solve the general case here, we claim correctness only for discrete locations at knot points. In that regard, we should note that a GC definition with a polyline main axis cannot provide a correct GC, since slope discontinuities at knot points create zero radius of curvature there.

The radius R_c of a cross section, $\vec{C}(t)$, is taken as the maximal distance of a point on its periphery, from its center:

$$R_c = \underset{t}{Max} \sqrt{C_x^2(t) + C_y^2(t)} \,, \qquad (F.2)$$

where $\vec{C}(t) = [C_x(t), C_y(t)]$ is the parametric vector representation of a cross-section curve. If the center point of the curve is located on the main axis curve, $\vec{A}(s)$, then the radius of curvature, $\rho(s)$, is

$$\rho = \rho(s) = (\dot{x}^2 + \dot{y}^2 + \dot{z}^2)^{3/2} / [\ (\dot{x} \cdot \ddot{y} - \dot{y} \cdot \ddot{x})^2 + (\dot{y} \cdot \ddot{z} - \dot{z} \cdot \ddot{y})^2 + (\dot{z} \cdot \ddot{x} - \dot{x} \cdot \ddot{z})^2\ ]^{1/2} \quad (F.3)$$

where

$$\dot{\alpha} = \frac{\partial}{\partial s} \alpha(s)$$

$$\ddot{\alpha} = \frac{\partial^2}{\partial s^2} \alpha(s)$$

for $\alpha = x, y, z$.

In general, $\dot{A} = \frac{\partial}{\partial s} \vec{A}(s)$, $\ddot{A} = \frac{\partial^2}{\partial s^2} \vec{A}(s)$, and both are vector functions of s:

$$\dot{A} = [\dot{x}, \dot{y}, \dot{z}]$$

$$\ddot{A} = [\ddot{x}, \ddot{y}, \ddot{z}] \,.$$

The mathematics leading to formula F.3 goes as follows ([Eisenhart, 1947]): if p is the natural parameter of the main axis curve, i.e., p corresponds to the curve's length, we define

$$A' = \frac{\partial}{\partial p} \vec{A}(p); \ A'' = \frac{\partial^2}{\partial p^2} \vec{A}(p) \qquad (F.4)$$

(Note: A' and A'' are vectors.)

Then: $\rho = \rho(p) = \dfrac{1}{|A''|}$,

where for some vector $\vec{\alpha}$, $|\vec{\alpha}|$ is its size, which is $\vec{\alpha} \cdot \vec{\alpha}$ with the vector dot product.

The relation between the natural parameter p and the given parameter s is some function ϕ

$$s = \phi(p) \tag{F.5}$$

that provides the following equations:

$$\frac{\partial s}{\partial p} = \frac{1}{\phi'} \quad \text{and} \quad \frac{\partial^2 s}{\partial p^2} = \frac{\phi''}{(\phi')^3}. \tag{F.6}$$

Now:

$$A' = \frac{\partial}{\partial s}\vec{A}(s) \cdot \frac{\partial s}{\partial p} = \dot{A} \cdot \frac{1}{\phi},$$

$$A'' = \frac{\partial^2}{\partial s^2}\vec{A}(s) \cdot \left(\frac{\partial s}{\partial p}\right)^2 + \frac{\partial}{\partial s}\vec{A}(s) \cdot \frac{\partial^2 s}{\partial p^2} \tag{F.7}$$

$$= \ddot{A}\,\frac{1}{(\phi')^2} - \dot{A} \cdot \cdot \frac{\phi''}{(\phi')^3}.$$

Also

$$\phi' = |\dot{A}|, \quad \phi' \cdot \phi'' = |\dot{A}| \cdot |\ddot{A}| \tag{F.8}$$

by F.5, F.6, and F.7:

$$A'' = \ddot{A} \cdot \frac{1}{|\dot{A}|^2} - \dot{A}\frac{(\dot{A} \cdot \ddot{A})}{|\dot{A}|^4} \tag{F.9}$$

$$\Rightarrow \rho = \frac{1}{|A''|} = \frac{|\dot{A}|^3}{\left[\ddot{A}^2 \cdot \dot{A}^2 - (\dot{A} \cdot \ddot{A})^2\right]^{1/2}}.$$

Eq. F.9 is equivalent to Eq. F.3 after some mathematical manipulations.

In the B-spline representation (see Appendix B), s varies between 0 and 1 at each segment of the main axis curve, so that at a given knot point, it is either 0 or 1, since that point is at one end of such a segment. To calculate ρ at such a point (e.g., $s = 0$), we have

$$\dot\alpha = [-3 \ 0 \ 3 \ 0] \ [V_\alpha]$$
$$\ddot\alpha = [3 \ -6 \ 3 \ 0] \ [V_\alpha] \qquad\qquad (\text{F.10})$$

for $\alpha = x,y,z$,

where $[V\alpha]$ is a 4-element coefficient column vector. Thus, if we define $[C] = [-3 \ 0 \ 3 \ 0]$, and $\ddot{C} = [3 \ -6 \ 3 \ 0]$, then

$$\dot\alpha \ \ddot\beta = [\dot{C}] \ [V_\alpha] \cdot [\ddot{C}] \cdot [V_\beta]$$
$$= [V_\alpha]^T \cdot [\dot{C}]^T \cdot [\ddot{C}] \ [V_\beta] \qquad\qquad (\text{F.11})$$
$$= [V_\alpha]^T \cdot [M] \cdot [V_\beta]$$

for $\alpha, \ \beta = x,y,z$

$$\dot\alpha^2 = [\dot{C}] \cdot [V_\alpha] \cdot [\dot{C}] \cdot [V_\alpha]$$
$$= [V_\alpha]^T \cdot [\dot{C}]^T \cdot [\dot{C}] \cdot [V_\alpha]$$
$$= [V_\alpha]^T \cdot [N] \cdot [V_\alpha]$$

for $\alpha = x,y,z$

and

$$[M] = \begin{bmatrix} -3 \\ 0 \\ 3 \\ 0 \end{bmatrix} [3 \ -6 \ 3 \ 0] = \begin{bmatrix} -9 & 18 & -9 & 0 \\ 0 & 0 & 0 & 0 \\ 0 & -18 & 0 & 0 \\ 0 & 0 & 0 & 0 \end{bmatrix}$$

$$\qquad\qquad (\text{F.12})$$

$$[N] = \begin{bmatrix} -3 \\ 0 \\ 3 \\ 0 \end{bmatrix} [3 \ 0 \ 3 \ 0] = \begin{bmatrix} -9 & 18 & -9 & 0 \\ 0 & 0 & 0 & 0 \\ 0 & -18 & 0 & 0 \\ 0 & 0 & 0 & 0 \end{bmatrix}$$

ρ is a function of $\vec{V}_\alpha$ ($\alpha = x,y,z$), which are coefficient vectors that depend on the geometric location of center points of cross sections. A given cross section will be banned from translating (i.e., moving its center-point location) if that will cause the appropriate to decrease below cross-section radius R_c: i.e.,

$$\rho > R_c \qquad\qquad (\text{F.13})$$

is the constraint formula.

Appendix G

Implementation Tools

G.1 SAIL and LEAP

SAIL is an ALGOL-like language [REISER, 1978], extended with sophisticated data types such as lists, sets, contexts, and procedure variables that are found in state-of-the-art programming languages. Unlike other languages, it contains the LEAP data structure that allows for the representation and manipulation of information networks, i.e., the creation and maintenance of complicated free-form data-bases. Two important elements of LEAP are *items* and *associations*. Items are considered nodes of networks whose links are represented by means of associations. The associative storage implemented in the language enables fast and efficient manipulation of and search for stored data.

Lists and sets are composed of items that are also the components of associations (termed *triples*). An item can be assigned any desired value of any legal data type in the language, including a procedure. Its value is accesssed via the language construct—Datum(*item, type*)—where *type* is redundant if the *item* is itself declared with some type. Items are treated like "constants"that are not bound to scope rules. The fact that items can contain anything makes it possible to maintain flexible and arbitrarily complicated data structure, although their being unbound to the lexical structure of the program puts the burden of storage management on the programmer. Multiprocessing and co-routines are also implemented through items; and procedural knowledge can be incorporated into networks by assigning procedures to node items. A thorough discussion with comparisons to other languages in the AI category is given by Bobrow [1974].

The contents of the associative store at any point in time can be selectively saved in files, and re-stored from them. This ability is useful in allowing the preparation of data structure by one program while the same data are being used by another. When a data structure is re-stored from a file, it may be desired to "link" some of the items from the file to others that are already in the associative store (i.e., the current "world"). This linking is accomplished through *PNAMES,* which are strings that represent a system-wide unique naming of items.

The syntax for associations is

$$\text{F } \textit{of } \text{O } \textit{is } \text{V,}$$

for example [FATHER *of* DAN *is* HENRY]. An association is created by the statement

$$\textit{make } \text{F } \textit{of } \text{O } \textit{is } \text{V.}$$

An item can be created in one of two ways, either by declaring it (limited, almost useless for large systems) or by creating *new* items as in:

$$\text{<item-var> := } \textit{new}(\text{ <expression> }),$$

which allocates a new item and assigns to it the type and value of <expression>. In essence, items and associations are represented in the same way, so that an association can also be part of yet other associations as one of the three associates thereof. Making associations is another way of allocating items.

Language constructs provide the tools to retrieve any element of an association, to find all items that are associated in some particular way, and to sequence through them in a repeating program block. The construct

$$\text{FATHER } \textit{of } \text{?WHO } \textit{is } \text{HENRY}$$

assigns to the item variable WHO, in some particular sequence, all items that are members of triples in which the first element is the item FATHER (or the contents of the item variable FATHER), and the third element is the item HENRY (or the contents of the item variable HENRY). The "?" before WHO is needed to allow *binding* that item-variable to retrieved items. For this purpose, WHO must contain the special item BINDIT prior to the invocation of this construct. Otherwise, such triples are merely predicates that will approve or deny the fact that something is in the associative store. To make this construct useful, it appears in iterative program blocks, i.e., *foreach* blocks. A foreach block can also sequence through sets and lists:

$$\textit{foreach } \text{<item var> } \textit{such that } \text{<item expression>}$$

$$\textit{do } \text{<block>.}$$

Yet another way to retrieve items from the associative store is by *derived sets* in which a second special item is introduced: the item ANY. The statement

fathers := FATHER *of* ANY

assigns to the set variable "fathers," all the items that are the third element of an association in which the first element is FATHER and the second one is anything, i.e., all those who have the FATHER relation with something.

Any of the allocated LEAP structures can be freed. Items are freed via the *delete* statement, while associations are *erase*-ed when the argument of the erasure statement is some particular association or a group of associations, that is accessed by using the item ANY. For example,

erase FATHER *of* ANY *is* HENRY

erases everything that associates HENRY as a FATHER of somebody. Note that erasing an association leaves the corresponding items alive.

The structure in Figure G.1 is expressed as

INSTANCE *of* G *is* N .

Figure G.1.   Graphical representation of "N is an instance of G."

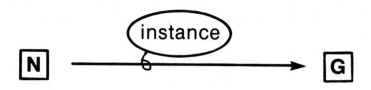

Each of the components of this association is an item. INSTANCE is a typeless item that has the system-wide unique *pname* INSTANCE. *G* is also such an item that deserves to be termed *generic,* of which *N* is an instance. In this case one may think of the item INSTANCE as a type of link between two nodes, one of which is a generic and the other is its instance. This link has a "direction" that is defined positionally; it can be traversed both ways, so that we can find all items that are INSTANCEs of something, or all those of which there is an INSTANCE, and so on.*

---

*NOTE

The key words *of* and *is* are usually referred to in SAIL manuals as "xor" and "eqv," respectively.

G.2 Representing DISTANCE in an Associative Network

G.2.1 General Discussion

An associative network is a declarative means to represent knowledge. This technique has two parts, the network itself, and an interpreter, which is a program that "knows" how to traverse the network and make sense out of it. To demonstrate this point and to solve a representational problem for the model, we shall compare several possibilities to represent the knowledge about the distance between two organs. The two organs L-Kidney and R-Kidney are items and are associated with all the information that concerns each of them individually. Two extremes are presented and compared. One puts most of the knowledge in a detailed network in which the meaning of links is represented in even more detailed associations via more items, turning the interpreter into a general-purpose program that can work on a large variety of networks. On the other hand, one can balance the representational power of the network by adding more knowledge to the interpreter, with the cost of turning it into a special-purpose program.

Following Brachman [Brachman, 1979] we represent the concept of DISTANCE as depicted graphically in Figure G.2. An instance of a DISTANCE is a structure similar to the concept definition. The various parts of a distance must correspond to the appropriate parts of the concept structure. Figure G.3 depicts the "individuation" of the concept DISTANCE as the geometric distance between the organs L-Kidney and R-Kidney.

Figure G.2.   Graphical representation of the concept DISTANCE by Brachman.

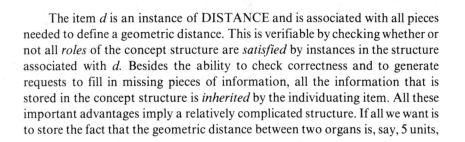

The item *d* is an instance of DISTANCE and is associated with all pieces needed to define a geometric distance. This is verifiable by checking whether or not all *roles* of the concept structure are *satisfied* by instances in the structure associated with *d*. Besides the ability to check correctness and to generate requests to fill in missing pieces of information, all the information that is stored in the concept structure is *inherited* by the individuating item. All these important advantages imply a relatively complicated structure. If all we want is to store the fact that the geometric distance between two organs is, say, 5 units,

Figure G.3. Graphical representation of the "individuation" of the concept DISTANCE to the instance of the geometric distance between two organs.

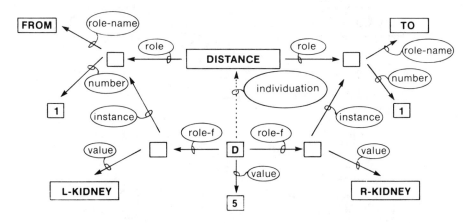

to be able to detect whether such information is recorded or not and to access it if possible, then the extra complexity is redundant. In general, we want to answer questions of this kind:

"What is the distance between L-Kidney and R-Kidney?"

or to carry out updates like

"Add 10 to the distance between L-Kidney and R-Kidney."

For this purpose, we have the knowledge as to what a distance is, stored in the program as a procedure; that is, there is a routine named Distance!Of(Organ1, Organ2), which can retrieve that knowledge from the model. In this case we can preserve space by storing the distance information as in Figure G.4. This representation views this kind of information as a property of the pair of organs involved. For relations of more than two organs, we have to talk about properties of more than two organs, and so on. We can talk about the item *neighbor* and refer to it explicitly (Figure G.4). A more general representation that will turn this link into a real node in the network, and so will be consistent with the network definition, is depicted in Figure G.5. The item N is associated with the two organs by the *role1* and *role2* links, and with its value via the *value* link. (We may primitivize the *role1* and *role2* links by representing them as instances of a generic node, ROLE, and signal their difference via a ROLE-NAME link. This way we are rapidly re-approaching Brachman's representation.)

Figure G.4.   Minimal representation of the distance between two organs.

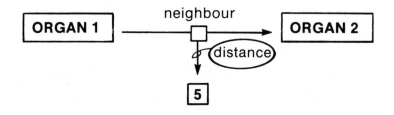

Figure G.5.   An associative network for the representation of the distance between two organs.

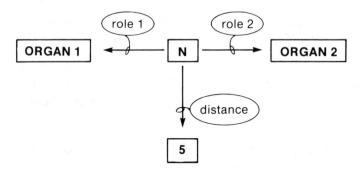

If there are some more pieces of information that concern these two organs, they can be added to the list of properties that these organs possess. Two ways to do so are depicted in Figure G.6. Here, we represent the distance and the predicative information that the two organs do not touch each other. Figure G.6A views every piece of information as another element in the property list of the two organs concerned. Figure G.6B views each new piece of information as a separate entity that has a special item to link it with the involved organs. In the method of Figure G.6B more items and associations are needed than in the method of Figure G.6A. As a matter of fact, if the number of properties to associate with a pair of organs is p, then the method of Figure G.6A will need $p+1$ extra items and $p+2$ extra associations. However, the method in Figure G.6B will need $2*p$ extra items and $3*p$ extra associations.

G.2.2 Information Generation

The representation as in Figure G.6A is more compact and is, moreover, a property list of the pair of organs involved. The representation in Figure G.6B allows us to talk about the class of DISTANCEs, or of the TOUCHINGs; it

Figure G.6.   Two ways to associate information pieces to a pair of
organs.

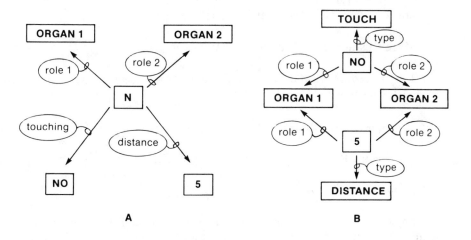

A   B

provides for a more efficient and faster search because of its use of greater
space. The SAIL code to create the association for the DISTANCE in Figure
G.6B is

```
itemvar X;
make TYPE of X:=new(5.) is DISTANCE;
make ROLE1 of X is Organ1;
make ROLE2 of x is Organ2;
```

For the representation of Figure G.6A, DISTANCE is represented with the aid
of a special link called *Neighborhood:*

```
real distance;
itemvar Neighborhood;
Neighborhood:= Neighborhood!Of(Organ1, Organ2);
distance:= if Organ1 of Neighborhood is Organ2
               then 5.0
               else —5.0;
make DISTANCE of Neighborhood is new(distance);
```

where the procedure Neighborhood!Of(Organ1, Organ2) checks whether
or not there is already a neighborhood relation between the two organ
items. If there is none, then the link will allocate and make the appropriate
item and association, and return the neighborhood item as its value. The
second statement is to check the "direction" of the neighborhood link,

since distance is relative to one organ or the other, and because we want to say that "the distance of Organ1 from Organ2 is 5 units."

In general and in any case, there will be a procedure (or a compile-time macro) that will generate these relations:

Make!Relation(organ1, organ2, relation-type, data):

This procedure will take care of the appropriate generations, as in the relations shown in Figure G.6B:

Make!Relation(Organ1, Organ2, DISTANCE, new(5.));

Make!Relation(Organ1, Organ2, TOUCHING, new(false)):

G.2.3 Information Retrieval

To complete the comparison, let's look at the amount of code that is needed to define the routine Distance!Of(Organ1, Organ2) for the retrieval of that information (see comments about the syntax at the end of this section).

For the representation in Figure G.3:

Algorithm G.1:

```
real procedure Distance(Organ1, Organ2);
 begin
  itemvar D,X,Y,V,Z;
  foreach D such that D is Individuation of DISTANCE do
    begin
      foreach X,Y such that (Role-F of D is X) and
                            (Role of X is Organ1) and
                            (Role-F of D is Y) and
                            (Role of Y is Organ2) do
    begin
      if (X is Instance of Z) and
        (Z is Role of DISTANCE) and
        (Y is Instance of V) and
        (V is Role of DISTANCE) then
      begin
          if (ROLENAME of Z is FROM) and
            (ROLENAME of V is TO) then
          return(VALUE of D);
          if (ROLENAME of Z is TO) and
```

```
            (ROLENAME of V is FROM) then
            return( -(VALUE of D));
      end
    end
  end
end;
```

For the representation in Figure G.6B:

Algorithm G.2:

```
real procedure Distance(Organ1, Organ2);
begin
  real itemvar D;
  foreach D such that (TYPE of D is DISTANCE) do
    begin
      if (ROLE1 of D is Organ1) and
         (ROLE2 of D is Organ2) then
         return (datum(D));
      if (ROLE1 of D is Organ2) and
         (ROLE2 of D is Organ1) then
         return (-datum(D));
    end
end;
```

for the representation in Figure G.6A.

Algorithm G.3:

```
real procedure Distance(Organ1, Organ2);
begin
  foreach N such that (N of Organ1 is Organ2) or
                      (N of Organ2 is Organ1) do
    begin
      if (N of Organ1 is Organ2) then
         return((DISTANCE of N))
      else return(-(Distance of N));
    end
end;
```

COMMENTS

1. While the representation in Figure G.5 is more detailed than the representation in Figure G.4, we use here a more compact form to represent a node, with the result that the statement

    (N *of* Organ1 *is* Organ2) in Algorithm G.3

is equivalent to having the two expressions

$$(ROLE1 \ of \ N \ is \ Organ1)$$

and

$$(ROLE2 \ of \ N \ is \ Organ2).$$

2. Retrieving a datum from an association is done somewhat differently from the method shown here: when the "DISTANCE *of* N" is needed, the appropriate syntax is

$$datum(\ lop \ (DISTANCE \ of \ N), \ real)$$

In general, compile-time macros will accomplish this task in the manner given for Distance!Of(N) in this example.

Appendix H

System Overview

The techniques presented in this study have been implemented as a software system on the DEC PDP10, under the TOPS10 operating system and in the programming language SAIL. The complete set of programs consists of tens of files and occupies about 300 pages of computer printout. When running, it uses about 100K of computer core for the code itself. The programs were written by the author during the two years in which the ideas and techniques were developed. These programs can be far more condensed and efficient in a second version.

Figure H.1 presents the main modules (files) of the system, some of which are additional supporting software packages. The system consists of three sets of modules that are named with the corresponding file names (six characters in the TOPS10 operating system of the DEC10 computer). The three major sets of files are summarized below:

1. *System:* Correspond to the hierarchical structure as depicted in Figure 3.1. *ModMat* is the top level, *OrgMdf,* and *Omatch* are the 'bag' of modifiers and matchers for the organ level, respectively; *SlcMdf* and *Smatch* are the corresponding experts for the cross-section level; and *BdrMdf* and *Bmatch* are for the boundary level.

2. *Utilities: Statis* are statistics utilities used at all levels to calculate results via the Selective-Mean (4.3.3); *3DIUtl* and *NTVpak* are the 3-D image utilities and a supporting package for the access of 3-D images; *SplInt, FSPUtl,* and *SplUtl* are three levels of utilities for the manipulations, definitions, display, and file storage for families of planar spline curves; *PCLrIn, FClUtl,* and *PClUtl* are for the definition, file storage, and generation of pseudocolors (by which most image figures in this dissertation were painted); *Blob* and *BSplin* are low-level packages that are used to manipulate spline curves at all system levels; *Orient* is a package that provides utilities for the geometrical interfaces between the hierarchical levels of the model and

the orientation of planar cross sections in a Generalized-Cylinder definition; *OrgUtl* are utilities for the definition and manipulation of organ components in the model; and Stblzr is a package that provides stabilizers for the converging of the iterative fitting process.

3. *Data:* Model definition is accomplished through a set of files. Each is a shape definition including all associated knowledge for the model of an organ at the cross-section level and below. Each of these files is named after its corresponding organ; all have extension *.SPL.* The higher levels of the model are defined by a SAIL program, *Model,* that uses the package *MakMod* for this purpose at initiation time. An alternative is a file of an already initiated and LEAP-dumped model definition.

The image is defined through a large set of RIFF files (2-D raster image files) and a structure that combines them into an integrated 3-D image of multiple resolutions. The combining structure is a file with extension *.IMG.*

Pseudocolors are stored in files with extension *.CLR.*

Figure H.1.   System overview: A block diagram of the system with respect to its program structure. Boxes in this figure are names of modules (files) of which the system and its data consist.

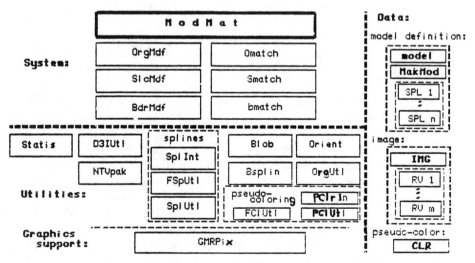

Figure H.2 presents a schematic of the major components and the data flow of the total system, including the provision of 3-D graphics display of the recovered anatomy. The *system* component (Figure H.1) takes a model and image-data for input and builds a model-instance that is a structure similar to the original model. Either of these structures (the model or its instance) may be fed to the surface-generation program, *Surface,* that builds a bilinear surface-representation for each of the organs in the model-instance. The *Graph* program displays this surface-representation in any desired form: wire-frame, shaded object, highlights, shadows, hidden lines, hidden surfaces, and so forth. Graphics are done on a Grinnell color raster graphics device model GMR26. An example of the expected results of this system is shown in Figure 1.4.

Figure H.2.   Major components and data flow diagram in which dashed boxes represent data structures which serve as input and output for the solid boxes that represent functional components and the graphics device.

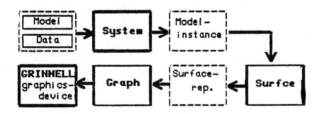

References

[Agin, 1972] Agin, G.J., "Representation and description of curved objects," Memo AIM-173, Stanford Artificial Intelligence Project (October 1972).

[Agin & Binford, 1976] Agin, G.J., and Binford, T.O., "Representation and description of curved objects," IEEE trans. on Computers, C-25, pp.440 (April 1976).

[Altschuler, 1979] Altschuler, M.D., et al., "Demonstration of a software package for the reconstruction of the dynamically changing structure of the human heart from cone-beam X-ray projections," Technical Report MIPG32, Department of Computer Science, State University of New York-Buffalo (1979).

[Badler, 1977] Badler, N.I., and O'Rourke, J., "A representation and display system for the human body and other 3-D curved objects," Technical Report, Computer Science Department, University of Pennsylvania (February 1977).

[Badler, 1978] Badler, N.I., and Bajcsy,R., "Three-dimensional representations for computer graphics and computer vision," Proceedings SIGGRAPH '78, pp.153-160 (August 1978).

[Ballard, 1978] Ballard, D.H., et al., "An Approach to Knowledge Directed Image Analysis," in Computer Vision Systems, Hanson, A.R., and Riesman, E.M. (eds.), Academic Press, pp.271-281 (1978).

[Ballard, 1980] Ballard, D.H., "Generalizing the Hough transform to detect arbitrary shapes," Technical Report 55, Computer Science Department, University of Rochester (October 1980).

[Ballard, 1982] Ballard, D.H. and Brown, C.M., Computer Vision, Prentice-Hall (1982).

[Birkhoff, 1956] Birkhoff, G.D., "On drawings composed of uniform straight lines," J. Math. Pures Appl. 19 (3), pp.793-754 (1940).

[Blum, 1964] Blum, H., "A transformation for extracting new descriptions of shape," Symposium on Models for Perception of Speech and Visual Form, Boston (November 1964).

[Bobrow, 1974] Bobrow, D., and Raphael, B., "New programming languages for AI research," ACM Computing Surveys 6(3), (September 1974).

[Bracewell, 1956] Bracewell, R.N., "Strip integration in radio astronomy," Aust. J. Phys. 9 (2), pp.198-217 (1956).

[Brachman, 1979] Brachman, R.J., "On the Epistemology Status of Semantic Networks," in Associative Networks, Findler, N.V. (ed.), Academic Press, pp.3-50 (1979).

[Brooks, 1975] Brooks, R.A., and DiChiro, G., "Theoryofimage reconstruction in computed tomography," Radiology 117, pp.561-572 (December 1975).

[Brown, 1979] Brown, C.M., "Fast display of well-tesselated surfaces," Technical Report 23, Computer Science Department, University of Rochester (1979).

[Ciarlet, 1975] Ciarlet, G.C., "Numerical Analysis of the Finite Element Method," Seminarde Mathematiques Superiores, Les Presses de L'Universite de Montreal (1975).

[Cohen, 1978] Cohen, P., Livingston R., and Summers, R. "Application programs for computer graphics: Dynamic view of CT image data," 16mm film, Roche Laboratories, Inc.and the Neuroscience Department, University of California-San Diego, La Jolla, California (1978).

(Available on video cassette: "The Brain: A Dynamic View of its Organization and Structure," by R.Livingston, from Roche Laboratories, Division of Hoffman-La Roche, Inc., Nutley, NJ 07110.)

[Coons, 1967] Coons, S.A., "Surface for Computer Aided Design of Space Forms," MAC-TR-41, Project MAC, Massachusetts Institute of Technology (June 1967).

[Crowther & Klug, 1971] Crowther, R.A., and Klug, A., "ART and science orconditions for 3-D reconstruction from electron microscope images," J. Theor. Biol. 32, pp.199-203 (1971).

[Curry & Schoenberg, 1947] Curry, H.B., and Schoenberg, I.J., "On spline distributions and their limits: the Polya distributions," Abst. Bull. Amer. Math. Soc. 53, pp.1114 (1947).

[DeBoor, 1972] DeBoor, C., "On Calculating with B-splines," J. Approx. Theory 6, pp.50-62 (1972).

[DeBoor, 1979] DeBoor, C., *A Practical Guide to Splines,* Springer-Verlag, 1979.

[DeRosier, 1971] DeRosier, D.J., "The reconstruction of three-dimensional images from electron micrographs," Contemp. Phys. 12 (5), pp.437-452 (1971).

[Dines, 1979] Dines, K.A., and Lytle, R.J., "Computerized geophysical tomography," Proc.IEEE special issue on Applications of Electromagnetic Theory to Geophysical Exploration 67:2(7), pp.1065-1073 (July 1979).

[Duda & Hart, 1973] Duda, R.O., and Hart, P.E., *Pattern Classification and Scene Analysis,* Wiley-Interscience (1973).

[Dwyer, 1983] Dwyer III, S.J., editor/chairman, Proceedings, 2nd International Conference and Workshop on Picture Archiving and Communication Systems (PACS II) For Medical Applications, SPIE Vol. 418, 303 pages (May 1983).

[Eisenhart, 1947] Eisenhart, L.P., *An Introduction to Differential Geometry with Use of the Tensor Calculus,* Princeton University Press, Chapter I, (1947).

[Findler, 1979] Findler, N.V. (ed.), *Associative Networks: Preparation and Use of Knowledge by Computers,* Academic Press (1979).

[Forrest, 1972]Forrest,A.R., "Interactive interpolation and approximation by Bezier polynomials," Comput. J. 15 (1), pp.71-79 (February 1972).

[Forrest, 1974] Forrest, A.R., "On Coons and other methods for the representation of curved surfaces," Comput. Graph. and Image Proc. 1, pp.341-359 (1974).

[Fuchs, 1977] Fuchs, H., Kedem, Z.M., and Uselton, S.P., "Optimal surface reconstruction from planar contours," Commun. ACM 20 (10), pp.693-702 (October 1977).

[Gilbert, 1972] Gilbert, P., "The reconstruction of three dimensional structurefromprojectionsand its applications to electron microscopy," II Direct Methods, Physical Society London, Proceedings, B 182, pp.89-102 (1972).

[Gilbert, 1972b] Gilbert, P., "Iterative Methods for the reconstruction of three-dimensional objects from projections," J. Theor. Biol. 36, pp.105-117 (1972).

[Goodenough, 1975] Goodenough, D.J., et al. "Potential artifacts associated with the scanning pattern of the EMI scanner," Radiology 117, pp.615-620 (December 1975).

[Gordon et al., 1970] Gordon, R., Bender, R., andHerman,G.T., "Algebraic reconstruction techniques (ART) for three-dimensional electron microscopy and X-ray photography," J. Theor. Biol.29, pp.471-481 (1970).

[Gordon, 1974] Gordon, R.and Herman, G.T., "Three dimensional reconstruction from projections: A review of algorithms," Inter. Rev. of Cyt. 38, pp.111-151 (1974).

[Gordon, 1975] Gordon, R., Herman, G.T., and Johnson, S.A., "Image reconstruction from projections," Sci. Am. 233, pp.56-68 (October 1975).

[Gouraud, 1971] Gouraud, H., "Computer display of curved surfaces," Technical Report UTEC-CSc-71-13, Computer Science Department, University of Utah (June 1971).

[Greenleaf, 1979] Greenleaf, J.F., Johnson, S.A., and Bahn, R.C., "Introduction to Computed Ultrasound Tomography," in *Computed Aided Tomography and Ultrasonics in Medicine,* Raviv et al.(eds.), North Holland Publishing Co. (1979).

[Hanson, 1976] Hanson, A.R., and Riesman, E.M., "Processing cones: A parallel computation of structure for scene analysis," COINS working paper, University of Massachusetts, Amherst (1976).

[Hanson, 1978] Hanson, A.R., and Riesman, E.M., "Vision: A computer system for interpreting scenes," in *Computer Vision,* Hanson, A.R.,and Riesman, E.M. (eds.), Academic Press, pp.303-334 (1978).

[Havlice, 1979] Havlice, J.F., and Taenzer, J.C., "Medical ultrasonic imaging: An overview of principles and instrumentation," Proc. IEEE special issue on Acoustic Imaging, 67:1(4), pp.620-641 (April 1979).

[Hering, 1961] Hering E., "Principles of a New Theory of Color Sense," in *Color Vision,* Teevan, R.C., and Birney, R.C. (eds.), D. Van Nastrand, Princeton, NJ (1961).

[Herman, 1978] Herman, G.T., and Liu, H.K., "Note: Dynamic boundary surface detection," Comput. Graph. Image Proc. 7, pp.130-138 (July 1978).

[Herman, 1979] Herman, G.T., and Liu, H.K. "Three dimensional display of human objects from computed tomograms," Comput. Graph. Image Proc. 9 (1), pp.1-21 (June 1979).

[Herman, 1980] Herman, G.T., *Image Reconstruction from Projections: The Fundamentals of Computerized Tomography,* Academic Press, New York (1980).

[Hinshaw, 1983] Hinshaw, W.S. and Lent, A.H., "An introduction to NMR imaging: from the Bloch equation to the imaging equation," Proceedings of the IEEE, Vol. 71(13), pp. 338-350 (March 1983).

[Hough, 1962] Hough, P.V.C., "Method and means for recognizing complex patterns," U.S. Patent 3,069,654 (December 18, 1962).

[Hounsfield, 1972] Hounsfield, G.N., "A method of and apparatus for examination of a body by radiation such as X- or gamma-radiation," British Patent 1283915, London (1972).(Issued to EMILtd. Application field, August 1968). Or: U.S. Patent 3,778,614 (1973).

[Huang, 1980] Huang, H.K., et al."Utilization of computerized tomographic scans as input to finite element analysis," International Conference Proceedings on Finite Elements in Biomechanics 2, pp.797-816 (February 1980).

[Hubel & Wiesel, 1962] Hubel, D.H., and Wiesel, T.N. "Receptive fields, binocular interaction and functions in the cat's visual cortex," J. Physiol. (London) 160, pp.106-154 (1962).

[Hueckel, 1969] Hueckel, M.H., "An operator which locates edges in digitized pictures," J. of the ACM 18 (1), pp.113-125 (January 1971).

[Klinger, 1979] Klinger, A., Rhodes, M.L., Kostanick, C., and Glenn, W.V., "General view imagery from orthogonal planes," Computer Science Department, University of Southern California.

[Kuhl & Edwards, 1963] Kuhl, D.E., and Edwards, R.Q., "Image separation radioisotope scanning," Radiology 80 (4), pp.653-662 (April 1963).

[Kuo, 1979] Kuo, Y.M., Glen, W.V. Jr., and Rhodes, M.L., "Elements of a comparative database for structure measurements in Computerized Tomography (CT)," Conf. on Computer Aided Analysis of Radiological Images, Newport Beach, CA (June 1979).

[Lemke, 1979] Lemke, H.U., Stiehl, H.S., Scharnweber, H., and Jackel, D., "Applications of picture processing, image analysis and computer graphics techniques to cranial CI scans," Proc., Sixth Conf. on Computer Applications in Radiology and Computer/Aided Analysis of Radiological Images, pp.341-354 (June 1979).

[Liu, 1977] Liu, H.K., "Two- and three dimensional boundary detection," Comput. Graph. Image Proc. 6, pp.123-134 (1977).

[Marr & Nishihara, 1976] Marr, D., and Nishihara, H.K., "Representation and recognition of a spatial organization of three dimensional shapes," A.I. Memo 377, Massachusetts Institute of Technology AI Laboratory (August 1976).

[Marr & Nishihara, 1977] Marr, D., and Nishihara,H.K., "Visual Information Processing: Artificial Intelligence and the Sensorium of Sight" (1977).

[Mategrano, 1977] Mategrano, V.C., et al., "Attenuation values in computed tomography of the abdomen," Radiology 125, pp.135-140 (1977).

[McCullough, 1976] McCullough, E.X., et al., "Performance evaluation and quality assurance of computed tomography scanners, with illustrations from the EMI, ACTA, and Delta scanners," Radiology 120, pp.173-186 (July 1976).

[McCullough, 1978] McCullough, E.C., and Payne J.T., "Patient dosage in computed tomography," Radiology 129, pp.457-463 (November 1978).

[Mueller, 1979] Mueller, R.K., Kaveh, M., and Wade, G., "Reconstructive tomography and application to ultrasonics," Proc. IEEE special issue on Acoustic Imaging, 67:1(4), pp.567-587 (April 1979).

[Natrella, 1963] Natrella, M.G., *Experimental Statistics,* National Bureau of Standards Handbook 91, U.S. Department of Commerce, Washington, D.C. (August, 1963).

[Newman, 1979] Newman W.M., Sproull, R.F., *Principles of Interactive Computer Graphics,* McGraw-Hill, 1979.

[Nevatia & Binford, 1977] Nevatia, R., and Binford, T.O., "Structured description of complexed objects," Artif. Intell. 8(6) (1977).

[Overhauser, 1968] Overhauser, A.W., "Analytic definition of curves and surfaces by parabolic blending," Technical Report SL 68-40, Scientific Research Staff, Scientific Laboratory, Ford Motor Company (May 1968).

[Plewes, 1980] Plewes, D.B., Violante, M.R., and Morris,T.W., "Intravenous Contrast Material and Tissue Enhancement in Computed Tomography," in *Medical Physics of CT and Ultrasound,* Fullerton, G.D., and Zagzebski, J.A., (ed.), published for the American Assoc. of Physicists in Medicine by the American Institute of Physics, pp.176-220 (1980).

[Poster, 1962] Poster, R.I., *Further Mathematics,* Bell and Sons, Ltd., London (1962).

[Radon, 1917] Radon, J., "On the determination of functions from their integrals along certain manifolds." (in German: "Ueber die bestimmung von Funktionen durch ichre integralwerte lungs gewisser Mannig-faltigkeiten"), Saechsische Ber. Verb. Saechs. Akademie Wiss., Leipzig, Math. Phys. Kl. 69, pp.262-277 (1917).

[Reiser, 1976] Reiser, J.F., et al., "SAIL," Stanford Artificial Intelligence Laboratory Memo AIM-289 (August 1976).

[Rhodes, 1979] Rhodes, M.L., "An algorithmic approach to controlling search in three-dimensional image data," Proceedings SIGGRAPH '79, pp.134-142 (August 1979).

[Riesenfeld, 1973] R. Riesenfeld, "Application of B-spline Approximation to Geometric Problems of Computer Aided Design," Ph.D. Thesis, Computer Science Department, Syracuse University (1973).

[Riteman, 1979] Riteman, E.L., Kinsey, J.H., Robb, R.A., Harris, L.D., and Gilbert, B.K., "Physics and technical considerations in the design of the dynamic spatial reconstructor (DSR— a high temporal resolution scanner)," SPIEJ.173, Application of Optical Instrumentation in Medicine VII, pp.382-390 (1979).

[Rubin, 1980] Rubin, S.M.,and Turner, W., "A3-dimensional representation for fast rendering of complex scenes," Proceedings SIGGRAPH '80, pp.110-116 (July 1980).

[Russell, 1979] Russell, D.M. "Where do I look now?" Proc.IEEE, Pattern recognition and image processing (August 1979).

[Samet, 1982] Samet, H., "Quadtrees and medial axis transform," Proceedings, 6th International Conference on Pattern Recognition, ICPR, pp. 184-187 (October, 1982).

[Schudy, 1980] Schudy, R.B., and Ballard, D.H., "Harmonic surfaces as models of biological objects," Ph.D. dissertation (in preparation), University of Rochester, Rochester, NY.

[Selfridge, 1979] Selfridge, P.G., and Sloan, K.R. Jr., "Raster image file format (RIFF): An approach to problems in image management," Pattern Recognition and Image Processing, pp.540-544 (August 1979).

[Shafer, 1983] Shafer, S.A. and Kanade, T., "The theory of straight homogeneous generalized cylinders and taxonomy of generalized cylinders," Technical Report CMU-CS-83-105, Department of Computer Science, Carnegie-Mellon University (January 1983).

[Sloan, 1977] Sloan K.R.Jr., "World model-driven scene analysis," Ph.D. dissertation, University of Pennsylvania (May 1977).

[Sloan & Bajcsy, 1977] Sloan, K.R. Jr., and Bajcsy, R., "World model driven recognition of natural scenes," Proc., Workshop on Picture Data Description and Management, pp.33-36 (April 1977).

[Soroka, 1979] Soroka, B.I., "Understanding objects from slices," Ph.D. dissertation, Technical Report TR-79-1, Department of Computer Science, University of Kansas (March 1979).

[Soroka, 1981] Soroka, B.I., Anderson, R.L. and Bajcsy, R.K., "Generalized cylinders from local aggregation of sections," Pattern Recognition, Vol. 13(5), pp. 353-363 (1981).

[Srihari, 1981] Srihari, S.N., "Representation of three dimensional digital images," Computer Surveys, Vol. 13(4), pp. 399-424 (December 1981).

[Srihary, 1982] Srihary, S.N., "Hierarchical data structures and progressive refinement of 3-D images," Proceedings, Pattern Recognition and Image Processing, PRIP'82, pp. 485-490 (June, 1982).

[Sunguroff, 1978] Sunguroff, A., and Greenberg, D., "Computer Generated images for medical applications," Proceedings SIGGRAPH'78, pp.196-202 (August 1978).

[Tanimoto, 1978] Tanimoto, S.L., "Regular Hierarchical Image and Processing Structures in Machine Vision," in *Computer Vision Systems,* Hanson, A.R., and Riesman, E.M. (eds.), Academic Press (1978).

[Tsai, 1976] Tsai, C.M., and Cho, Z.H., "Physics of contrast mechanism and averaging effect of linear attenuation coefficients in a computerized tranverse axial tomography (CTAT) transmission scanner," Phys. Med. Biol. 21(4), pp.544-559 (1976).

[Winston, 1977] Winston, P.H., *Artificial Intelligence,* Addison Wesley (1977).

[Wu, 1977] Wu, S., Abel, J.F., and Greenberg, D.P., "An interactive computer graphics approach to surface representation," Comm. ACM 20(10), pp.703-712 (October 1977).

[Voelcker, 1978] Voelcker, H., et al. "The PADL-1.0 /2 system for defining and displaying solid objects," Proceedings SIGGRAPH '78, pp.257-263 (August 1978).

[Yamaguchi, 1978] Yamaguchi, F., "A New Curve-Fitting Method Using a CRT Computer Display," (a note), Computer Graphics and Image Processing 7, pp.425-437 (1978).

[Zucker, 1979] Zucker, S.W., and Hummel, R.A., "An optimal three-dimensional edge operator," Report No. 79-10, Computer Vision and Graphics Laboratory, McGill University (April 1979).

Index